1001 MULTIPLE CHOICE QUESTIONS AND ANSWERS IN SURGERY

1001 Multiple Choice Questions and Answers in Surgery

based on

Bailey and Love's 'Short Practice of Surgery'
(Edited by Rains and Ritchie)

BY

A. J. HARDING RAINS, M.S., F.R.C.S.

Professor of Surgery, University of London
Honorary Consultant, Charing Cross Hospital, London

(With an additional 101 Questions and Answers on Surgical History)

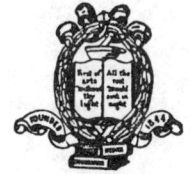

LONDON
H. K. LEWIS & CO. LTD
1978

First Published 1978

©
1978
H. K. Lewis & Co. Ltd

This book is copyright.
It may not be reproduced by any means
in whole or in part without permission.
Applications regarding copyright
should be addressed to the Publishers.

ISBN 0 7186 0439 3

PRINTED IN GREAT BRITAIN
FOR H. K. LEWIS AND CO. LTD
BY HAZELL WATSON AND VINEY LTD, AYLESBURY, BUCKS

MULTIPLE CHOICE QUESTIONS (M.C.Q.)
and how to use this book

Here are questions for anyone who studies surgery. The questions are suitable for those at every stage – for the first-year student, for the student preparing for 'finals' and for the postgraduate embarking upon a career in surgery which includes the hurdles of postgraduate degrees and diplomas.

Multiple choice questions appear in several guises when they are used to test understanding and factual knowledge across the whole field of education outside as well as inside medicine. But in the testing of surgical knowledge in particular two types are generally popular: (a) the single response (1 in 4, or 1 in 5) and (b) the determinate response ('Yes' and 'No'). Both types of question start off with a main reference to a problem which sets the scene and this is called the 'stem'.

Below the stem are set out the various options available as answers.

Single Response. In the single correct response type of question (the 1 in 4 or 1 in 5 style) you are presented with either 4 or 5 options. One answer is correct and is called the 'key'. Naturally the other and incorrect options are called distractors.

For example:

Stem = An uncomplicated inguinal hernia
Option A   has an expansile impulse on coughing
Option B   is irreducible
Option C   does not descend into the scrotum
Option D   transilluminates

A is obviously the single correct response (the key). B, C, D are incorrect distractors.

Occasionally the questioner will give you a clear directive 'Which of .... is correct?'. He may however ask 'Which of the .... is incorrect?'.

He might ask you to decide whether the whole question; stem and option is one which requires a single positive response or is one which is inverted and requires a single negative response. Certainly this 'inversion' forces you to give careful and equal consideration to each option rather than just spotting the single 'Yes'. You will discover that I have included some 'inversions' in Parts I and III. There are nearly

90 of them in Part I and you will find that they are identified by an asterisk.

To avoid becoming confused it is often helpful to read the stem before each option (or even better to say it quietly to yourself), for example:

Stem = The disadvantages of internal fixation of a fractured shaft of femur include
    A. stiffness of the knee. ? Agree ? Disagree

Stem = The disadvantages of internal fixation of a fractured shaft of femur include
    B. the impossibility of reduction due to the interposition of soft parts. ? Agree ? Disagree

Stem = The disadvantages of internal fixation of a fractured shaft of femur include
    C. prolonged treatment in hospital. ? Agree ? Disagree

Stem = The disadvantages of internal fixation of a fractured shaft of femur include
    D. the complication of osteomyelitis. ? Agree ? Disagree

You have disagreed with A, B and C and agreed with D. D is the key which fits the stem. D is the 1 in 4, and the single correct positive response.

Conversely and contrariwise if the questioner should set an 'inversion', the 'key' is the option which is 'No, I disagree' and the other answers are 'Yes, I agree' – for example:

Stem = In Simmonds' disease there is
    A. destruction of the posterior lobe of the pituitary. ? Agree ? Disagree

Stem = In Simmonds' disease there is
    B. Amenorrhoea. ? Agree ? Disagree

Stem = In Simmonds' disease there is
    C. atrophy of the skin. ? Agree ? Disagree

Stem = In Simmonds' disease there is
    D. wasting from anorexia. ? Agree ? Disagree

You should have disagreed with A and agreed with B, C and D. So A is the single negative response.

Also I would draw your attention to the use by some scheming examiners of what amounts to a double negative between the stem and the key. See option C of the first example just given or this:

Stem = Basophil adenomas of the pituitary are not
    A. inconsiderable in size.

You would agree that these adenomas are normally inconsiderable (*i.e.* small) in size so you would disagree with the stem and option when put together, which is tantamount to saying they are large. The main reason for inserting one or two of these 'twisters' amongst the questions that follow is to train you to read questions carefully and answer what is asked. Failure to do this is nothing short of disaster in any part of the examination.

The Determinate Type of M.C.Q. This type has become very popular in examinations, and is very suitable for testing medical and surgical knowledge and judgement. There are usually five options to test either agreement or disagreement with the stem and you have to determine which of the options to say 'Yes' to and which to say 'No' to. You are required, if possible, to commit yourself because you are given a mark for correct 'No' as well as for correct 'Yes' responses. Also with most systems you lose a mark for an incorrect response but do not lose a mark if you decline to respond. Thus if you give all correct responses in a question you score $+5$, but if you give all incorrect responses you score -5, and if you do not attempt any you score 0! Needless to say there are some questions in which the answers to all the options is 'Yes' and some in which the answers are all 'No'.

About the Questions in this Booklet

They have been prepared not only to test you but also to assist you in covering the whole ground of surgery as presented in clinical practice and in a textbook such as the 'Short Practice'. Naturally they should be of assistance in revision and in clearing up points of uncertainty.

The questions are presented in four parts. The first two parts are questions which are serial in relation to the chapters in 'Short Practice', Part One being the single response 1 in 4 type and Part Two being the determinate type. In this way the questions and answers can easily be checked against the text and it is hoped that further reading (and reading around the subject) will be stimulated if necessary. Part Three (1 in 4) and Part Four (determinate) are questions set at random and, therefore, are akin to the examination scene. However it is quite a simple matter to check with and read around chapter and verse. In Part Three the questions are presented in short related runs, as this is a feature of some styles of M.C.Q. examinations. Part Four begins like this also, but changes to complete randomisation in order to make things that much more difficult. It is hoped that by extending you in this way the booklet will be completing its purpose.

But having said a great deal about stems, keys, options and distractors, I should also point out that some of the questions are addressed to a subject in a general way and that the options are not options but a series of questions in themselves. This is a device used by some to widen the scope of testing in a particular subject. In the context of this booklet it is also a device to encourage wide initial coverage of a particular subject as well as wide revision.

About Practising M.C.Q.

There is no doubt at all that practising M.C.Q. before an examination makes a difference to your performance on the day. Indeed those who do not practise now find themselves at a disadvantage. Furthermore it is very necessary for those who find M.C.Q. difficult, distressing and generally distasteful to persevere.

Sometimes the satisfactory performance of a student in the clinical and oral parts of an examination is irretrievably marred by a disaster in the M.C.Q. The way to prevent this happening is to practise.

About Pretested Questions and the Suitability of these Questions to all Grades of Ability

When multiple choice questions are devised for examination purposes it is essential that the options offered are effective in discriminating between the good and the bad candidates. A question that is too easy or an option which is too obvious is valueless, and so is a question or option which is too difficult for all (in spite of the fondness with which an examiner cherishes it). Therefore, for a particular examination a bank of questions is built up of those with options which have been tested previously in medical school classes or in an examination. A computer is used to determine which are valuable and which are useless discriminators.

About Performance in this Booklet

In the stems, keys, options and distractors presented are many that have been tested in final examinations. However, because the booklet is designed to suit everyone from entry to maturity in clinical work, I have deliberately introduced some very easy and some relatively difficult questions. But all should attempt all. The first-year clinical student might achieve a 20–30% success rate (I hope more), the final student a 40–60% success rate and the postgraduate studying, say, for the F.R.C.S. or a Mastership 70–100%. I am reminded of my student days when a great surgical teacher on a ward round always posed the same questions to the assembled nurses, clinical students, Fellowship and Mastership postgraduates with some very surprising results!

About M.C.Q. in General

We can be quite certain that the M.C.Q part of an examination has come to stay. It has become a useful adjunct to any kind of assessment of factual knowledge, but it has not in the minds of most examiners proved itself, as was first hoped, superior to the essay or short written answer. We hear much debate about whether the M.C.Q. can test understanding and attitudes as well as factual knowledge, about those ambiguities of experience in clinical practice which, of necessity, creep so easily into the M.C.Q. options with words like 'often', 'generally', 'usually', 'may', *etc.*, and about marking systems, raw scores and percentiles. Indeed M.C.Q. invites continuous debate, polemics and histrionics and is a happy hunting ground for the medical educationalists. One is often reminded of the stanza from the 'Rubaiyat of Omar Khayyam' with which readers from all over the world are familiar –

> *Myself when young did eagerly frequent*
> *Doctor and Saint, and heard great argument*
> *About it and about : but evermore*
> *Came out by the same door as in I went.*

Suffice to say again that M.C.Q. is here to stay and, therefore, the best thing to do is to practise and to use it in such a booklet as this, to assist in the study and revision of the principles and practice of surgery as experienced at the bedside and in the operating theatre, and as set out in the text book.

March 1978   A. J. HARDING RAINS

CONTENTS

PART I.	Single Response (1 in 4) in Series Questions 1–300	1
PART II.	Determinate Response (Yes and No) in Series Questions 301–600	49
PART III.	Single Response (1 in 4) Set at Random Questions 601–800	111
PART IV.	Determinate Response (Yes and No) Set at Random. Questions 801–1001	145
PART V.	Historical – Single Response (1 in 4) in Series Questions 1–101	189
ANSWERS.	Parts I–V	209

PART I
SINGLE RESPONSE (1 IN 4) IN SERIES

Note: It is suggested that if you wish to mark the options you use a soft graphite pencil and not any other writing instrument. In an examination you are given a pencil with which to mark the answer form (a) because usually if a computer is doing the marking it picks up your response *via* the graphite in the pencil and (b) because you can easily rub out and alter a response. In this booklet also you can rub out the responses and start afresh at any time.

Remember that most questions require a single correct (Yes) response. Those requiring a single incorrect response (No) are identified by an asterisk.

PART I

1. **The best dressing is**
   A skin
   B scab
   C gauze and bandage
   D Aerosol plastic spray

2. **Healing by first intention means**
   A using catgut
   B obtaining union between two edges of an incision without subsequent breakdown
   C the immediate use of a plastic dressing
   D the method whereby an ulcer heals

3. **Debridement of a wound means**
   A excising 1 mm skin from the edges of a wound
   B not excising skin but excising all damaged muscle
   C laying open and therefore unleashing all layers of a wound
   D delayed primary suture

4. **'Butcher's thigh' implies**
   A hypertrophy of the thigh muscles in butchers due to humping meat
   B rupture of muscles due to humping meat
   C bursa of the femoral triangle
   D division of one of the femoral vessels of a butcher when a boning-knife slips

5. **The 'second accident' is**
   A further trauma to the body occurring seconds after the primary trauma
   B a fatality due to imperfectly sustained first aid
   C another accident due to the same cause of the first accident
   D accidental injury to another person by the first person who is injured

6. **The extent of muscle damage by a bullet depends principally upon**
   A size
   B velocity
   C shape
   D weight

7. **An antibioma is**
   A   an all powerful antibiotic
   B   an antibiotic contaminant
   C   a malignant tumour caused by an antibiotic
   D   an excess mass of fibrous tissue around a small abscess persistently treated by antibiotics

8. **Cellulitis is**
   A   inflammation of the bone marrow
   B   inflammation of the mastoid air cells
   C   inflammation of the subcutaneous tissues
   D   infiltration of the skin by giant cells

9. **A foaming liver is a complication of**
   A   hydatid disease
   B   gas gangrene
   C   portal pyaemia
   D   cirrhosis

10. **A malignant pustule is**
    A   an infected secondary deposit in the skin
    B   a rapidly spreading rodent ulcer
    C   an infected molluscum sebaceum
    D   anthrax of the skin

11. **One of the following is an acute specific infection**
    A   Diphtheria
    B   Actinomycosis
    C   Tuberculosis
    D   Leprosy

12. **TNM classification of a malignant tumour was designed as**
    A   an histological staging
    B   a clinical staging
    C   a staging carried out at operation
    D   a staging dependent upon radio scanning and skeletal survey

13. **What is known as a 'recurrent fibroid' occurs in**
    A   an ovarian cyst
    B   the uterus
    C   a scar
    D   the jaw

14. **An hydatid cyst is, in origin**
    A congenital
    B bacterial
    C neoplastic
    D parasitic

15. **Which of the following is not a worm?**
    A Taenia solium
    B Taenia coli
    C Taenia saginata
    D Taenia echinococcus

16. **The term 'ulcer' is, by definition**
    A an erosion of the skin
    B a discontinuity of any epithelial surface
    C a lesion always caused by infection
    D a neoplastic process

17. **Eusol is a**
    A solution of Eugenol
    B solution derived from boric acid and bleaching powder
    C saline intravenous solution designed for the European Common Market
    D a type of carbolic acid

18. **Dermatitis artefacta is**
    A due to nickel sensitivity
    B due to arsenic sensitivity
    C self-induced
    D doctor-induced

19. **The floor of a tuberculous ulcer will be seen to contain**
    A apple jelly granulations
    B a wash-leather slough
    C strawberry granulations
    D fat

20. **A blue-green discharge from an ulcer indicates infection with**
    A pseudomonas pyocyaneus
    B streptococcus viridans
    C candida albicans
    D staphylococcus aureus

21. **Oriental sore is due to**
    A a protozoal infection
    B a guinea worm
    C a bamboo splinter
    D sand

22. **Secondary haemorrhage occurs**
    A within 6 hours of operation
    B 7–14 days after operation
    C as a result of violent coughing on recovery from anaesthesia
    D due to a blood transfusion line being disconnected

23. **The percentage of the circulating blood volume in the venous system and splanchnic vessels is normally between**
    A 20–30%
    B 40–50%
    C 60–70%
    D none of these

24. **After haemorrhage lost plasma proteins are replaced by**
    A the small intestine
    B the liver
    C the spleen
    D the muscles

25. **Morphine given for injury is primarily**
    A a sedative
    B an analgesic
    C a diaphoretic
    D an emetic

26. **Packed red cells are prepared by**
    A filtration
    B centrifugation
    C freeze-drying
    D precipitation

27. **In an acute emergency if blood has to be given immediately without full laboratory cross-matching it is best to give blood which is**
    A Group O RhD −ve
    B Group O RhD +ve
    C Group AB RhD −ve
    D Group AB RhD +ve

28. **Mannitol is**
    A a type of sugar
    B a type of dextran
    C a type of lipid for i.v. feeding
    D contraindicated in the treatment of shock

29. **The minimum urine output for 24 hours required to excrete end products of protein metabolism is**
    A 200 ml
    B 300 ml
    C 400 ml
    D 500 ml

30. **The total body sodium amounts to**
    A 2500 mmol
    B 5000 mmol
    C 7500 mmol
    D 10000 mmol

31. **The percentage of potassium in the extracellular fluid is**
    A 2%
    B 10%
    C 20%
    D 25%

32. **Potassium deficiency is present if the plasma-potassium level is less than**
    A 5·0 mmol/l
    B 4·5 mmol/l
    C 4·0 mmol/l
    D 3·5 mmol/l

33. **There is a danger in giving saline intravenously when it is made up as**
    A chemically normal saline
    B isotonic saline
    C 0·9%
    D 0·18% with Dextrose 4·3%

34. **Which of the following veins should be avoided in adults, if possible, for intravenous infusion?**
    A Median vein of the forearm
    B Cephalic
    C Long saphenous
    D External jugular

35. **Proctoclysis is**
    A a cryo-operation for piles
    B dilatation of the anus
    C Rectal biopsy
    D giving water and electrolytes per rectum

36. **Parenterovite is**
    A a high calorie intravenous fluid
    B a type of intravenous lipid for parenteral nutrition
    C a vitamin injection
    D a vitamin capsule for oral ingestion

37. **The standard bicarbonate level in the plasma is normally**
    A 12–15 mEq/l
    B 16–21 mEq/l
    C 22–25 mmol/l
    D 26–31 mmol/l

38. **In health the pH of the blood lies between the range**
    A pH 7·05–7·19
    B 7·20–7·35
    C 7·36–7·44
    D 7·45–7·59

39. **In health the ratio of bicarbonate to carbonic acid is normally**
    A 10:1
    B 15:1
    C 20:1
    D 30:1

40. **The daily minimum protein intake necessary to keep a healthy adult in positive nitrogen balance is**
    A 25–30 g
    B 35–40 g
    C 45–50 g
    D 55–60 g

41. **Elemental or 'space' diets alone are not used for patients with**
    A intestinal fistula
    B short bowel syndrome
    C malabsorption states
    D diverticulosis

42. **Lupus vulgaris is**
    - A a generalised collagen disease
    - B a local collagen disease of the face
    - C a syphilitic lesion on the face
    - D a tuberculous lesion on the face

43. **A boil is**
    - A any abscess of the skin
    - B the same as a carbuncle
    - C an acute infection of a hair follicle
    - D an infection of a hair follicle by demodex folliculorum

44. **A molluscum sebaceum is otherwise known as**
    - A a seborrhoeic wart
    - B dermatofibroma
    - C a keratoacanthoma
    - D a benign calcifying epithelioma

45. **A rhinophyma is**
    - A a sebaceous cyst of the nose
    - B a rodent ulcer of the nose
    - C a glandular form of acne rosacea
    - D a nasal form of Boeck's sarcoid

46. **A port wine stain (Naevus flammeus) is**
    - A a premalignant lesion of the skin
    - B a type of melanoma
    - C a type of bruising of the skin
    - D a type of haemangioma

47. **A strawberry angioma in a baby should be treated by**
    - A cryosurgery
    - B radiotherapy
    - C excision
    - D masterly inactivity

48. **A rodent ulcer is**
    - A a squamous cell carcinoma
    - B a basal cell carcinoma
    - C only occurs on the face
    - D contains epithelial pearls

49. **A Wolfe graft is**
    A a partial thickness skin graft
    B a pinch skin graft
    C a small full thickness skin graft
    D a pedicle graft

50. **A dermatome is**
    A an area of skin supplied by the branch of a particular nerve
    B a type of comb used for cleaning infected hair
    C a machine for cutting a full thickness skin graft
    D an opening in the skin made for a colostomy

51. **'Rest pain' occurs**
    A anywhere in the body at rest
    B in the thigh of a patient with Buerger's disease
    C in the calf of a patient with intermittent claudication
    D in the foot of a patient with severe vascular disease

52. **Harvey's sign is**
    A loss of hair from the toes in peripheral vascular disease
    B distended veins in the foot in spite of arterial occlusion
    C gauging the speed of venous return by emptying a length of vein
    D transmitted pressure wave on coughing in severe varicose veins

53. **A Seldinger needle is used for**
    A liver biopsy
    B suturing skin
    C arteriography
    D lymphography

54. **A useful though temporary improvement in a patient's ischaemic foot can be attained by giving intravenously**
    A 10% Mannitol
    B 10% Dextrose
    C Dextran 40
    D Dextran 100

55. **Lumbar sympathectomy is of value in the management of**
    A intermittent claudication
    B distal ischaemia affecting the skin of the toes
    C arteriovenous fistula
    D diabetic neuropathy

56. In arterial by-pass surgery the best vein to use is
    A the cephalic
    B the femoral
    C the long saphenous
    D the short saphenous

57. Today the commonest cause of a true aneurysm is
    A congenital
    B syphilitic
    C atherosclerosis
    D a gunshot wound

58. Which is the correct spelling?
    A Absess
    B Abcess
    C Abscess
    D Abses

59. Nicoladoni's sign is also known as
    A Harvey's sign
    B Grey turner's sign
    C Murphy's sign
    D Branham's sign

60. An overdose of Heparin is treated by
    A prostaglandins
    B phenidione
    C protamine sulphate
    D prostigmine

61. Thromboendarterectomy is
    A the ideal operation for Buerger's disease
    B the ideal operation for Raynaud's disease
    C used for carotid artery stenosis
    D the same operation as embolectomy

62. Buerger's disease is
    A due to atherosclerosis
    B an obliterative arteritis of young females
    C confined to Ashkanazy Jews
    D often associated with attacks of thrombophlebitis

63. **Sympathectomy is not advised for**
    A Raynaud's disease of the fingers
    B hyperhidrosis of the feet
    C intermittent claudication
    D acrocyanosis

64. **A sequestrum is**
    A a piece of soft dead tissue
    B a piece of dead skin
    C a dead tooth
    D a piece of dead bone

65. **A decubitus ulcer is**
    A a venous ulcer
    B an ulcer in the region of the elbow
    C a pressure sore
    D an ulcer of the tongue

66. **Trench foot is**
    A sodden infected skin of the foot following the digging of a trench in wet weather
    B an ischaemic condition of the foot following exposure to damp and cold in tight footwear
    C gas gangrene of the foot
    D chilblains of the toes

67. **The term 'venous pump' refers to**
    A the apparatus used for rapid transfusion of blood
    B part of autotransfusion apparatus
    C musculofascial anatomy and physiology of the calf
    D the presence of valves in the inferior vena cava

68. **Clinically a saphena varix is most likely to be confused with**
    A Baker's cyst
    B femoral hernia
    C a spermatocoele
    D a soft sore

69. **The Brodie-Trendelenberg test is used to detect**
    A the presence of deep femoral vein thrombosis
    B the integrity of the long saphenous nerve
    C the presence of an incompetent valve at the saphenofemoral junction
    D the presence of an incompetent valve at the junction of the short saphenous and popliteal veins

70. Operations for varicose veins are best accomplished by
    A stripping
    B multiple subcutaneous ligatures
    C subfascial ligatures
    D division and ligation at the sites of a bad leak from the deep to the superficial venous system

71. The appropriate management of thrombophlebitis of superficial veins is
    A supportive bandages and ambulation
    B supportive bandages and strict bed rest
    C anticoagulants and bed rest
    D anticoagulants and ambulation

72. Acute lymphangitis of the arm requires
    A no special treatment
    B immediate multiple incisions
    C immediate lymphangiogram
    D an immediate systemic antibiotic

73. Milroy's disease is lymphoedema
    A which follows filariasis
    B which is familial
    C which follows erysipelas
    D which is the sequel to white leg

74. The cisterna chyli are situated
    A in the pelvis
    B in the thorax
    C in the posterior cranial fossa
    D in the abdomen

75. A cystic hygroma is
    A a type of hydrocoele
    B a type of lymphangioma
    C a type of branchial cyst
    D a cystic sweat gland tumour

76. Which of the following is not related to the histological appearance of Hodgkin's disease?
    A Langhans giant cells
    B Reed-Sternberg cells
    C Eosinophils
    D Reticulum cells

13

77. The five-year cure rate for lymphosarcoma after modern treatment is
    A 30%
    B 50%
    C 70%
    D 85%

78. A patient presenting with a pulp abscess of the finger should be treated principally with
    A penicillin
    B chloramphenicol
    C incision
    D poulticing

79. Which of the following is not applicable to Boeck's sarcoidosis?
    A Kveim test
    B Potaba (potassium-p-amino-benzoate)
    C Corticosteroid therapy
    D Casoni test

80. In some 80% of cases of infection of the hand the organism is
    A gram negative bacillus
    B *streptococcus pyogenes*
    C *staphylococcus aureus*
    D a clostridium

81. When performing primary treatment of untidy hand injuries it is essential
    A to obtain skin closure
    B to repair divided nerves
    C to repair divided tendons
    D to repair divided tendons and nerves

82. The maximum safe time that a tourniquet may be left on for the purpose of obtaining a bloodless field in hand surgery is (should not exceed)
    A 45 minutes
    B one hour
    C one hour 30 minutes
    D two hours

83. One of the following is not the eponym associated with the operation for ingrowing toenail:
    A Quenu
    B Zadik
    C Fowler
    D Girdlestone

84. A Gigli saw is
    A an electrically driven circular bone saw
    B a pneumatically driven bone saw
    C a short straight bone saw
    D a long twisted wire bone saw

85. Which of the following terms is inappropriate to the condition osteomyelitis?
    A Cloacae
    B Involucrum
    C Sequestrum
    D Myelocoele

86. A Brodie's abscess is
    A a subperiosteal abscess due to infection of the mastoid air cells
    B a type of breast abscess
    C a chronic abscess of the bone
    D an abscess arising in the inguinal lymph nodes

87. Pott's disease is
    A a fracture dislocation about the ankle
    B a neuropathic joint
    C traumatic osteochondritis of the spine
    D tuberculosis of the spine

88. 'Melon seed' bodies are found in
    A the peritoneal cavity following pancreatitis
    B a bunion
    C a compound palmar ganglion
    D the bladder in tuberculous cystitis

89. The initial abnormality in primary osteoarthrosis is
    A in the synovial membrane
    B sclerosis of cartilage
    C fibrillation of cartilage
    D an osteophyte

90. **Still's disease is**
    A spastic diplegia
    B rheumatoid arthritis in childhood
    C rheumatoid arthritis in the elderly
    D post-traumatic bone formation in the lateral ligament of the knee

91. **Which one of the following operations is inappropriate in the treatment of osteoarthrosis?**
    A Synovectomy
    B Arthrodesis
    C Arthroplasty
    D Osteotomy

92. **A benign tumour forming osteoid is**
    A a synovioma
    B a chondroma
    C an osteoma
    D a fibroma

93. **Which of these statements are incorrect concerning chondrosarcoma?**
    A It occurs mainly in middle-aged persons
    B It is rare in children
    C It has a predilection for flat bones
    D It does not metastasise to the lung

94. **The most reliable method of obtaining a biopsy of a bone tumour is by means of**
    A a Trucut needle
    B a drill
    C open operation
    D a Menghini needle

95. **Ewing's tumour of bone**
    A should be locally excised
    B should be treated by immediate amputation
    C looks like a cut onion on x-ray
    D has a soap-bubble appearance on x-ray

96. **Barlow's sign is related to the diagnosis of**
    A talipes equinus varus
    B congenital dislocation of the hip
    C ulnar nerve palsy
    D genu varum

97. **Trendelenburg's sign is used in the diagnosis of**
    A varicose veins
    B congenital dislocation of the hip
    C carcinoma of the stomach
    D pulmonary embolism

98. **The word talipes refers to**
    A long feet with spidery toes
    B club feet
    C flat feet
    D hammer toes

99. **Bone dysplasia is due to**
    A faulty nutrition
    B faulty development
    C parathyroid tumour
    D trauma

100. **Idiopathic scoliosis is a**
    A lateral curvature of the spine
    B rotation of the spine
    C lateral curvature with rotation of the spine
    D flexion deformity of the spine

101. **The Risser turnbuckle cast is used to**
    A correct deformity occurring in the union of a fracture
    B correct kyphosis
    C overcome fixed flexion of the hip joint
    D correct scoliosis

102. **Legg-Calve-Perthe's disease is**
    A osteochondritis of the spine
    B tuberculosis of the hip joint
    C slipped proximal femoral epiphysis
    D osteochondritis of the proximal femoral epiphysis

103. **Dead bone is recognised on x-ray because**
    A it is more radiolucent than normal
    B it is more radiopaque
    C osteophytes grow out around it
    D it has a soap-bubble appearance

104. **Paget's disease of bones is synonymous with**
 A osteitis deformans
 B osteitis fibrosa cystica
 C osteomalacia
 D osteopetrosis

105. **Osteogenic sarcoma develops in Paget's disease in**
 A 1% of patients
 B 5% of patients
 C 15% of patients
 D none

106. **Osteoclasis can be used to**
 A correct deformity of the tibia due to rickets
 B curette an osteoclastoma
 C correct deformity due to Paget's disease
 D correct a ricketed rosary

107. **Adrenocorticosteroids in excess cause**
 A osteoporosis
 B osteosclerosis
 C osteochondritis
 D endochondral ossification

108. **Tennis elbow is**
 A olecranon bursitis
 B 'non-articular rheumatism' of the extensor muscles of the forearm to the lateral epicondyle of the humerus
 C 'non-articular rheumatism' of the attachment of the flexor muscles to the medial epicondyle
 D myositis ossificans of the supinator muscle

109. **In Dupuytren's contracture which one of the following statements is incorrect?**
 A It is a contracture of the flexor tendons to the ring and little fingers
 B It is a contracture of the palmar fascia
 C It may occur in the plantar fascia
 D There is an association with cirrhosis of the liver

110. **A Baker's cyst is**
    A   an implantation dermoid cyst occurring in the palms of those who work in a bakery
    B   a synovial cyst of the wrists of those who work in a bakery
    C   a synovial cyst of the popliteal fossa
    D   a synovial cyst of the ankle

111. **Which of the following is incompatible with the effects of an ulnar nerve palsy?**
    A   Anaesthesia over the hypothenar eminence
    B   Anaesthesia over the anatomical snuff box
    C   A positive Froment's sign
    D   Hyperextension of the 4th and 5th metacarpophalangeal joints

112. **Metatarsus primus varus is a cause of**
    A   pes cavus
    B   talipes equinovarus
    C   hallux varus
    D   hallux valgus

113. **Hammer toes**
    A   do not develop adventitious bursaa
    B   are due to injury caused by a heavy object (*e.g.* a hammer) falling on the toes
    C   can be treated by the spike arthrodesis operation
    D   should not be amputated

114. **Plantar fasciitis**
    A   is caused by a bony spur on the plantar surface of the os calcis
    B   is not associated with infection elsewhere in the body
    C   is a type of Dupuytren's disease
    D   can be relieved by supplying insoles

115. **Union of a simple transverse fracture of the tibia in an adult normally takes**
    A   6 weeks
    B   8 weeks
    C   12 weeks
    D   18 weeks

116. **Which type of fracture does not impact?**
    A Fracture of the vault of the skull
    B A compression fracture
    C A simple fracture
    D A traction injury

117. **Which of the following is not a definite cause of delayed union of a fracture?**
    A Shear
    B Infection
    C Bending
    D Systemic disease

118. **In an adult patient with a fracture of the shaft of the femur**
    A no blood can be lost without obvious swelling
    B no blood can be lost without obvious bruising
    C two litres of blood can be lost without obvious swelling or bruising
    D There is no likelihood of death from haemorrhagic shock

119. **A plaster of Paris splint used to immobilise a fracture should**
    A immobilise the joints above and below the fracture
    B not immobilise any joint below the fracture
    C be applied dry and then sprayed with water
    D always be put on and left for 48 hours completely surrounding the affected limb

120. **A plaster of Paris spica is**
    A a metal footpiece incorporated in the plaster for weight bearing
    B a plaster bandage used for avulsion fractures of the terminal phalanx of a finger
    C a plaster bandage around the pelvis and upper thigh with a resulting pattern that resembles an ear of wheat
    D a metal pin which is used for traction purposes of a plaster cast

121. **A Colles' fracture is**
    A common in adolescence
    B a fracture about the ankle joint
    C common in elderly women
    D a fracture of the head of the radius

122. **In the treatment of fractures of both forearm bones in a child, which of the following is unacceptable?**
    A   Closed manipulation
    B   A residual angulation of 5°
    C   Onlay plates
    D   Rush nails

123. **Regarding supracondylar fracture of the humerus in children which of the following is correct?**
    A   It is due to a fall on the point of the elbow
    B   It is usually compound
    C   Admission to hospital is essential following reduction
    D   It requires open reduction

124. **A fracture of the clavicle is best treated by**
    A   clavicle rings
    B   a figure of eight bandage
    C   open reduction and plating
    D   a sling and analgesics

125. **A Pott's fracture is a type of fracture of**
    A   the wrist
    B   the ankle
    C   the spine
    D   the foot

126. **A comminuted fracture of the patella should be treated by**
    A   physiotherapy alone
    B   removal of the smallest fragments
    C   removal of all the patella
    D   inserting screws or wire

127. **Concerning fractures of the neck of the femur which statement is considered now to be incorrect?**
    A   It is common in elderly women
    B   It can occur in young adults due to fatigue
    C   It can occur in young adults following severe violence applied in the long axis of the femur
    D   The bone fractures in an elderly woman because she falls

128. In the management of an unconscious patient with a head injury which of the following is incorrect?
    A The patient should not be secluded in a darkened room
    B An x-ray of the skull is unnecessary
    C The patient should not be nursed in the supine position
    D The patient should be turned regularly

129. In head injuries which substance is not included in therapy?
    A Urea
    B Mannitol
    C Dexamethazone
    D Hyaluronidase

130. Of the clinical features of chronic subdural haemorrhage which of the following statements is incorrect?
    A There is always a preceding loss of consciousness
    B There can be severe headache
    C There is slowness of response to questions
    D Stupor may come and go

131. Regarding meningiomas which of the following is incorrect?
    A They include endotheliomas
    B They are usually flat
    C They cause reactive hyperostosis
    D About 18% of intracranial tumours are meningiomas

*132. Craniopharyngiomas
    A are calcified in 50% of cases
    B are removable
    C form large masses
    D have cystic cavities

*133. Congenital hydrocephalus is often associated with
    A myelomeningocoele
    B the Arnold-Chiari malformation
    C failure of development of the arachnoid villi
    D a cerebral tumour

134. **Below the level of the lesion in spinal concussion (produced by long axis stretch on the cord accompanying flexion) there is (with one exception)**
    A a flaccid paralysis
    B retention of urine
    C loss of joint sense
    D loss of pain and temperature sensation

135. **In the immediate management of a patient who may possibly have a cervical spine injury, which of the following statements is incorrect?**
    A Cervical injuries should be transported with the head lifted on to a pillow
    B The patient should be left lying on the stretcher until examination is completed
    C If a cord lesion is present the best immediate examination is testing the sensory level to pinprick on the trunk
    D A lateral x-ray should be taken without disturbing the patient

136. **In spondylolisthesis which statement is incorrect?**
    A The forward displacement of the vertebral body does not narrow the spinal cord
    B A congenital defect in the development of the pedicles is the likely cause
    C Most patients require lumbosacral fusion
    D The deformity can cause root pressure and sciatica

137. **A Bell's palsy is a paralysis affecting the**
    A fifth cranial nerve
    B seventh cranial nerve
    C eighth cranial nerve
    D serratus anterior muscle

138. **A Klumpke paralysis includes all except one of the following:**
    A It is a lower brachial plexus lesion
    B There is wasting of the thenar muscles only
    C There is sensory loss along the inner side of the forearm
    D There is sensory loss of the inner three and a half fingers

139. **A 'Saturday night' palsy is**
    A temporary lower limb paralysis due to alcoholic intoxication
    B acute retention of urine
    C injury to the radial nerve in the radial groove
    D anaesthesia of the tongue

140. **Froment's sign is a test for**
    A median nerve palsy
    B foot drop
    C wrist drop
    D ulnar nerve palsy

141. **Regarding orbital cellulitis, which of the following is incorrect?**
    A It is a common complication of acute sinusitis
    B Enophthalmos is present
    C Intensive antibiotic therapy is required initially
    D The sinusitis may require surgical drainage

142. **An hyphaema is**
    A lymphoedema of the face
    B a type of cat-bite on the face
    C haemorrhage into the frontal sinus
    D blood in the anterior chamber of the eye

143. **The aim of treatment of an infant with a cleft lip is to**
    A improve appearances
    B make feeding possible
    C achieve adequate speech
    D achieve adequate dentition

144. **Tumours of the palate include the following except**
    A ectopic salivary tumour
    B a carcinoma of the maxillary antrum
    C an alveolar abscess of the incisors
    D a transitional-cell carcinoma

145. **Countryman's lip is**
    A swelling due to sensitivity to the sun
    B an early lesion of foot and mouth disease
    C a squamous-cell carcinoma
    D a mucous cyst of the lip

146. **Fracture of the nasal bones may be reduced by one of the following:**
    A Moynihan's forceps
    B Lion forceps
    C Walsham's forceps
    D MacIndoe's forceps

147. A dental cyst
- A contains an unerupted incisor tooth
- B contains an unerupted molar tooth
- C occurs in connection with the root of an erupted normal tooth
- D occurs in connection with the root of an erupted but chronically infected tooth

148. Epiphora is
- A an epiphenomenon of a cerebral tumour
- B cerebrospinal fluid running from the nose after a fracture of the anterior fossa
- C an abnormal overflow of tears due to obstruction of the lacrymal duct
- D eversion of the lower eyelid following injury

149. A deflected nasal septum is treated by
- A inserting a prosthesis
- B removal
- C straightening
- D submucous resection

150. Regarding acute mastoiditis, which of the following is incorrect?
- A There is periauricular swelling
- B The pinna is very painful on movement
- C There is conductive deafness
- D Pus must be let out

151. Which is not a complication of chronic otitis media?
- A Presbyacusis
- B Facial palsy
- C Labyrinthitis
- D Conductive deafness

152. Ménière's disease can be treated by
- A a plastic operation
- B a prosthesis
- C stapedectomy
- D labyrinthectomy

153. **Regarding aphthous stomatitis which of the following is incorrect?**
    A It is confined to infants
    B It can be due to a virus
    C It can be caused by Monilia
    D It can be caused by Candida

154. **A ranula is a**
    A cystic swelling in the floor of the mouth
    B forked uvula
    C sublingual thyroid
    D thyroglossal cyst

155. **Leukoplakia of the tongue is not associated with**
    A a jagged tooth
    B smoking
    C dyskeratosis
    D aspergillus niger

156. **In carcinoma of the tongue which of the following is incorrect?**
    A It is virtually symptomless in its early stages
    B One form of presentation is a fissure
    C It may cause earache
    D The usual site is the back of the tongue

157. **The Commando operation is**
    A abdomino-perineal excision of the rectum for carcinoma
    B disarticulation of the hip for gas gangrene of the leg
    C extended radical mastectomy
    D excision of carcinoma of the tongue, the floor of the mouth, part of the jaw and lymph nodes *en bloc*

158. **Which of the following is incorrect regarding the thyroid?**
    A The gland develops from the third pharyngeal pouch
    B The C-cells are developed from the ultimo-branchial body
    C The normal gland weight 20–25g
    D The resting follicle contains colloid in which iodine is stored

159. **Long-acting thyroid stimulator is**
    A a glycoprotein
    B di-iodothyronine
    C an Ig M immunoglobulin
    D an Ig G immunoglobulin

160. **In simple nodular goitre**
   A carcinoma occurs in 30% of cases
   B The nodular stage is irreversible
   C operation is contraindicated
   D the patient does not develop hyperthyroidism

161. **Regarding the clinical solitary nodule of the thyroid which statement is incorrect?**
   A The solitary toxic nodule is never malignant
   B The solitary toxic nodule may be treated by radio cobalt
   C The 'cold' nodule is suspect (*i.e.* may be malignant)
   D The 'cold' nodule should be excised

162. **The Caldwell-Luc operation is**
   A for removing nasal polypi
   B for cataract
   C for draining intractable purulent maxillary sinusitis
   D for closing an oral-antral fistula

163. **Vincent's angina is a form of angina associated with**
   A spasm of the oesophagus
   B diphtheria
   C an infection of the mouth
   D coronary artery spasm

164. **Acanthosis is**
   A an inflammation of the inner canthus of the eye
   B a proliferation of the prickle cell layer
   C a rodent ulcer of the inner canthus of the eye
   D leukoplakia of the anus

165. **The Pes Anserinus is**
   A syndactyly affecting the toes
   B club foot
   C the arrangement of the cervical plexus in the neck
   D a description of the arrangement of the facial nerve

166. **The treatment of submandibular calculus lying within the duct is to**
   A dilate the duct
   B remove the stone by making an opening in the duct
   C slit open the duct at the papilla
   D remove the gland

167. **A Warthin's tumour is**
    A   an adenolymphoma of the parotid gland
    B   a pleomorphic adenoma of the parotid
    C   a cylindroma
    D   a carcinoma of the parotid

*168. **A branchial cyst**
    A   arises from the second branchial cleft
    B   usually appears between the ages of 20–25 years
    C   protrudes beneath the anterior border of the sternomastoid
    D   is always lined by squamous epithelium

169. **Which of the following is inappropriate to cystic hygroma?**
    A   It is a type of cavernous haemangioma
    B   It can be the earliest swelling of the neck to appear in life
    C   It can obstruct labour
    D   It is brilliantly translucent

170. **The 'potato' tumour of the neck is a**
    A   sternomastoid tumour
    B   carotid body tumour
    C   thyroid tumour
    D   parotid tumour

171. **Which of the following is incorrect about exophthalmos?**
    A   It is always bilateral
    B   In severe cases corneal ulceration may occur
    C   Hypothyroidism may make it worse
    D   There is widening of the palpebral fissure

172. **Which of the following is not an antithyroid drug?**
    A   Carbimazole
    B   Propranolol
    C   Propyl-thiouracil
    D   Potassium perchlorate

173. **Which of the following is used in the treatment of a thyrotoxic crisis?**
    A   Propranolol
    B   Metaclopramide
    C   Tetraiodophenolphthalein
    D   Radio-iodine

174. Which of the following is not an histological type of carcinoma of the thyroid?
    A Transitional
    B Papillary
    C Anaplastic
    D Medullary

175. Hashimoto's disease is
    A a granulomatous thyroiditis
    B an auto-immune thyroiditis
    C an infiltrating fibrosis of the thyroid and the adjacent muscles
    D focal thyroiditis

176. A thyroglossal fistula
    A is never congenital
    B follows inadequate removal of a thyroglossal cyst
    C has a hood of skin with its concavity upwards
    D is lined by squamous epithelium

177. Regarding the parathyroid glands, they
    A are normally two in number
    B lie inside the capsule of the thyroid
    C are reddish-blue in colour
    D are not the secretors of calcitonin

178. Chvostek's sign is
    A carpal spasm induced by sphygmomanometer cuff pressure on the upper arm above the systolic blood pressure for not more than two minutes in the normal person
    B as above, but the person has tetanus
    C twitching of the facial muscles produced by tapping over the branches of the facial nerve at the angle of the jaw in the normal person
    D as above, but the person has tetany

179. After operation for hyperparathyroidism which of the following does not take place?
    A Renal stones disappear
    B Bones recalcify
    C Psychiatric patients improve
    D Hyperparathyroidism recurs in a small minority of patients

180. **Concerning the adrenal glands, which of the following is incorrect?**
   A The adrenal glands have attained nearly adult proportions at birth
   B The right adrenal is semilunar in shape
   C On the left side the adrenal vein enters into the left renal vein
   D The left gland is a little larger than the right

181. **Regarding the Waterhouse-Friderichsen syndrome:**
   A Most cases occur in adults
   B Treatment should await the result of blood culture
   C Adrenalectomy is indicated
   D It is a complication of meningitis

182. **In Cushing's syndrome**
   A There is chronic hypocorticism
   B There is an excessive production of glucocorticoids
   C There is a malignant adrenal neoplasm present in about 50% of cases
   D One third of the patients have a basophil tumour of the adrenal

*183. **Regarding phaeochromocytoma:**
   A It is bilateral in about 15% of cases
   B It produces noradrenaline
   C All patients under 60 years who present with sustained arterial hypertension deserve a routine test to confirm or exclude the condition
   D Treatment should depend upon antihypertensive drugs

184. **Which is the incorrect statement about the lymphatic system draining the breast?**
   A There is a free communication between the subclavicular and supraclavicular lymph nodes
   B The lymph nodes along the internal mammary chain are involved in about half the cases in which the axillary nodes are implicated by carcinoma
   C The thoracic chain of lymph nodes lie along the internal mammary vessels
   D Some lymph nodes lie between the greater and lesser pectoral muscles

185. **A cracked nipple is**
    A   due to a syphilitic chancre
    B   a cause of a retention cyst of a gland of Montgomery
    C   Paget's disease of the nipple
    D   a forerunner of a breast abscess

186. **A blood-stained discharge from the nipple means that the patient may have**
    A   papilloma of the nipple
    B   fibroadenoma
    C   duct papilloma
    D   duct ectasia

187. **A breast lump is safe to leave alone after aspiration if**
    A   it is a cyst which does not subsequently refill
    B   it is solid and not cystic
    C   there is minimal bloodstaining of the aspirate
    D   cytological examination reveals cells with hyperchromatic nuclei

*188. **Massive swellings of the breast include the following:**
    A   Cystosarcoma phylloides
    B   Atrophic scirrhous carcinoma
    C   Diffuse hypertrophy
    D   Giant fibroadenoma

189. **The following are clinical signs supporting an early diagnosis of carcinoma of the breast:**
    A   A prickling sensation in a breast lump
    B   *Peau d'orange*
    C   Brawny arm
    D   Cancer *en Cuirasse*

*190. **Regarding follow-up of patients with carcinoma of the breast:**
    A   It is unnecessary for a surgeon to follow-up his patients with carcinoma of the breast after operation. It is done by other specialties
    B   A rectal examination may be necessary
    C   The liver should be examined
    D   X-ray of the chest is a routine follow-up examination

191. **The usual cause of acute follicular tonsillitis is**
    A *streptococcus pyogenes*
    B *staphylococcus aureus*
    C *klebsiella*
    D candidiasis

*192. **Regarding a pharyngeal pouch:**
    A It protrudes through Killian's dehiscence
    B It usually turns to the left side of the neck
    C It may be visible in the neck
    D It is twice as common in boys as in girls

193. **A malignant tumour in the sinus piriformis**
    A often presents first as an enlarged lymph node behind the angle of the jaw
    B causes pain in the hip
    C causes pain in the hand
    D commonly presents with pain in the area concerned

*194. **Cytotoxic agents used in the treatment of malignant disease include**
    A nitrogen mustard
    B epoxy resins
    C methotrexate
    D vinka alkaloids

195. **Which one of the following is not a cause of acute oedema of the glottis?**
    A Ludwig's angina
    B Angioneurotic oedema
    C Hot steam
    D Leukoplakia

196. **A cricoid hook is used particularly**
    A in thyroidectomy
    B in block dissection of the neck
    C for retracting the superior laryngeal nerve
    D in tracheostomy

*197. **Papilloma of the larynx**
    A is relatively common in childhood
    B is the commonest benign tumour of the larynx
    C often becomes malignant
    D the symptoms are similar to those of carcinoma of the larynx

*198. **Segments of the right lung include the**
   A upper lobe
   B middle lobe
   C the lingular segments
   D the lower lobe

*199. **Isolated rib fractures**
   A are painful
   B are shown clearly on x-ray
   C may be treated by analgesics
   D may require intercostal nerve block

*200. **A pneumothorax**
   A is the presence of air between the pleura and the rib cage
   B can be spontaneous
   C has the physical signs of a hyperresonant percussion note with absent breath sounds
   D can be recurrent

*201. **An empyema**
   A is never primary
   B is preceded usually by a serous effusion
   C if due to pneumococcal infection contains a great deal of fibrin
   D should be drained immediately by rib resection and underwater seal drain

*202. **Benign tumours of the lung include**
   A adenoma
   B hamartoma
   C carcinoid adenoma
   D mesothelioma

*203. **The histological types of carcinoma of the bronchus are**
   A round cell
   B squamous cell
   C columnar cell
   D transitional cell

*204. **Carcinoma of the bronchus**
   A is suspected in a patient with unresolved 'pneumonia'
   B commonly presents with haemoptysis
   C can present with secondary deposits in the brain
   D is suspected if there is neuropathy without chest symptoms

*205. **Lung cysts may be**
   A pseudo-cysts
   B epithelial cysts
   C parasitic cysts
   D adenolymphomatous cysts

*206. **Post-operative pulmonary complications are largely predisposed to by**
   A smoking
   B pain
   C lack of mobility
   D the anaesthetic

207. **Pulmonary embolism**
   A is not limited to surgical wards
   B usually follows superficial thrombophlebitis
   C is mostly a paradoxical embolism
   D is an acceptable cause of 5% of all hospital deaths

208. **Regarding eventration of the diaphragm, which statement is irrelevant?**
   A It is due to defective development
   B Symptoms are uncommon
   C Volvulus of the stomach may occur
   D There is a defect between the sternal and costal attachments

*209. **Anterior mediastinal tumours include**
   A retrosternal goitre
   B teratoma
   C neurofibroma
   D pleuropericardial cyst

*210. **Factors leading to cardiac arrest include**
   A obstruction to the airway
   B inhalation of fresh water
   C excess of potassium
   D excess of calcium

*211. **In a patent ductus arteriosus**
   A the pressure in the aorta is higher than in the pulmonary artery
   B the ductus connects with the right pulmonary artery
   C as much as 10–20 litres of blood per minute can flow through a patent ductus
   D There is a water hammer pulse

*212. An atrial septal defect
- A causes overfilling of the left side of the heart
- B produces a pulmonary systolic murmur
- C may cause little disability in childhood
- D can be closed by direct suture under direct vision

*213. If an aorto-coronary by-pass graft is performed
- A the main indication is angina which cannot be controlled by medical means
- B coronary arteriography must show a blocked or stenosed coronary artery with a normal vessel beyond
- C lengths of femoral vein are used to by-pass a narrowed artery
- D 80–90% can obtain relief from angina

*214. Dysphagia
- A is the term used to describe pain on swallowing
- B may be oropharyngeal and oesophageal
- C may be for solids or liquids
- D may be vague in its appreciation

215. The sign of oesophageal atresia is
- A the newborn baby regurgitates all its first feed
- B the abdomen becomes distended
- C saliva pours almost continuously from the mouth
- D attacks of coughing on feeding

*216. The cardiac sphincter
- A can be demonstrated anatomically
- B is manifest as a zone of high intraluminal pressure
- C is maintained by valvular effects of the oesophagogastric angle
- D is maintained by 'rosette-like' folds of the gastric mucous membrane

*217. Hiatus hernia should be operated upon
- A as soon as one course of medical treatment has failed
- B if there is oesophageal stenosis
- C by using the abdominal approach as a rule
- D by employing the Nissen fundoplication procedure

218. Cardiospasm is
- A due to coronary atheroma
- B due to coronary spasm
- C due to presbyoesophagus (corkscrew oesophagus)
- D a functional obstruction of the oesophagus

*219. **The diagnosis of carcinoma of the lower third of the oesophagus can be made by**
   A oesophagoscopy
   B biopsy
   C mediastinoscopy
   D exfoliative cytology

220. **The gastroduodenal artery is a branch of the**
   A coeliac axis
   B hepatic artery
   C superior mesenteric artery
   D gastroepiploic artery

*221. **The parietal cells of the stomach**
   A lie in the gastric crypts of the body of the stomach
   B are about one billion in number in a normal adult male
   C are about four billion in Zollinger-Ellison syndrome
   D are the chief cells of the stomach

*222. **Current tests of gastric secretion include**
   A a test meal
   B night fasting secretion
   C maximal acid output
   D insulin test

223. **Regarding hypertrophic pyloric stenosis which statement is correct?**
   A The cause is unknown
   B The musculature of the pyloric antrum is atrophied
   C Firstborn female infants are most commonly affected
   D In 50% of cases it is the father who bears the scar of an operation for this condition in infancy

*224. **Regarding chronic gastric ulcers:**
   A The patients are often blood group O
   B They tend to occur in alkaline mucosa
   C The muscularis mucosae tends to be fused with the muscularis at the edge of the ulcer
   D Epithelial proliferation and downgrowths indicate malignant change

*225. **The essentials of the conservative management of an acute exacerbation of a peptic ulcer include**
    A no smoking
    B bed rest
    C regular meals
    D soluble aspirin for pain

*226. **Regarding a perforated peptic ulcer:**
    A It is most frequently situated on the lesser curve of the stomach
    B It is more common in men
    C The highest incidence is between 45–55 years
    D A perforated gastric ulcer could well be malignant

227. **Regarding pyloric stenosis, which statement is incorrect?**
    A It may be due to a carcinoma at or near the pylorus
    B It is due to cicatrisation from a duodenal or pyloric gastric ulcer
    C It occurs usually in men with a long history of ulcer symptoms
    D A succussion splash can be heard

*228. **Regarding gastrocolic fistula:**
    A The patient does not usually present by vomiting faeces
    B It should be suspected when a patient with a gastro-enterostomy has sudden severe diarrhoea
    C The patient is troubled by diarrhoea after every meal
    D The gastric contents pass directly into the colon

*229. **The undesirable effects of vagotomy include**
    A diarrhoea
    B loss of gastric motility producing distension
    C gastric ulceration
    D iron-deficiency anaemia

230. **In connection with carcinoma of the stomach, which of the following is incorrect?**
    A Anaemia
    B A negative test for occult blood
    C Raised sedimentation rate
    D Achlorhydria or hypochlorhydria

*231. **Post-operative acute dilatation of the stomach is suggested by**
   A hiccoughs and rising pulse rate
   B effortless vomit
   C dark watery vomit
   D considerable flatus

*232. **The functions of the spleen are**
   A to provide 500 ml of blood to add to the circulation in case of haemorrhage
   B to destroy effete erythrocytes
   C to produce antibodies
   D to form erythrocytes and lymphocytes

*233. **Regarding ruptured spleen:**
   A It occurs easily in infectious mononucleosis
   B It can be caused by a fall
   C The usual clinical features are: Initial shock, recovery from shock, signs of a ruptured spleen
   D Kehr's sign of pain in the right shoulder may be present

*234. **Purpura**
   A is a cause of intussusception
   B is a cause of haematuria
   C can appear as large bruised areas
   D is confirmed by the appearance of petechiae after a sphygmomanometer cuff is inflated above the systolic pressure for ten minutes

*235. **Regarding liver biopsy:**
   A It can be performed on any patient
   B It can be performed with a Menghini needle
   C Tumours can be missed
   D The puncture can be performed in the epigastrium

236. **Which of the following is not associated with cirrhosis of the liver?**
   A Gynaecomasia
   B Testicular atrophy
   C Pale palms
   D Dupuytren's contracture

*237. A secondary deposit in the liver
  A is umbilicated
  B can be confidently diagnosed by palpation at laparotomy
  C can be treated by resection
  D can come from a primary melanoma in the eye

*238. Cholecystography
  A is essential in the diagnosis of chronic gallbladder disease
  B is valueless if the patient is jaundiced with a plasma bilirubin level of over 3 mg/100 ml
  C is not contra-indicated if the renal function is impaired
  D can also show up the hepatic and common bile ducts

*239. Peroperative cholangiography
  A reveals the presence of gallstones in the common hepatic duct
  B confirms the anatomy of the ducts
  C confirms the patency of the duodenal papilla
  D confirms the anatomy of the arterial supply to the gallbladder and liver

240. Gallstones do not contain
  A protein
  B phosphate
  C carbonate
  D oxalate

*241. Mixed gallstones
  A in size are generally concretions of no more than 5 mm down to sludge particles
  B can contain salmonella
  C constitute the majority of gallstones
  D may be faceted

242. The usual treatment of gallstones in the common ducts is
  A cholecystostomy
  B choledochoduodenostomy
  C sphincterotomy (of the duodenal papilla)
  D cholecystectomy and choledochotomy

*243. Carcinoma of the gallbladder
  A accounts for 10% of all malignant neoplasms
  B is in 90% of cases associated with the presence of gallstones
  C may begin by squamous metaplasia
  D carries a dismal prognosis (2% surviving five years)

*244. Mucoviscidosis of the pancreas
   A is acquired
   B affects the lungs
   C causes meconium ileus
   D affects the sweat glands

*245. The treatment of acute pancreatitis
   A should be conservative if there is any doubt about the diagnosis
   B includes the use of atropine or propantheline
   C may include calcium gluconate intravenously
   D may include large doses of antibiotics

*246. Carcinoma of the pancreas
   A occurs mostly in the head of the gland
   B is associated with a distended gallbladder in 60% of cases
   C may cause the passage of 'aluminium' stools
   D is not related to diabetes

247. In generalised peritonitis
   A the patient rolls around in agony
   B morphine or pethidine (demerol U.S.P.) is useful while the patient is under observation
   C the patient lies still
   D the pulse rate falls progressively

248. The clinical features of a mesenteric cyst include, with one exception, the following:
   A It may be a painless abdominal swelling
   B It causes recurrent attacks of abdominal pain
   C It moves freely in the long axis of the mesentery
   D It may present as an acute abdomen

*249. Retroperitoneal tumours include
   A ganglioneuroma
   B lipoma
   C sarcoma
   D enterogenous cyst

*250. **In traumatic rupture of the small intestine from whatever cause**
- A it is liable to occur in the presence of an irreducible inguinal hernia
- B the mucosa prolapses in small perforations and tends partially to seal the rent
- C injury to the duodenojejunal junction is easily overlooked
- D the mesentery usually escapes injury

*251. **Meckel's diverticulum**
- A is present in 2% of the human race
- B in 90% of cases arises from the mesenteric border of the ileum
- C may contain heterotopic pancreas
- D occurs with equal frequency in both sexes

*252. **Diverticular disease is not**
- A restricted to the sigmoid colon
- B unknown in Africans
- C related to the sites where blood vessels penetrate the bowel wall
- D precancerous

*253. **Regarding ulcerative colitis:**
- A The cause is unknown
- B The disease starts in the rectum and spreads proximally in 95% of cases
- C There may be a 'sea' of ulceration
- D Pain is the usual earliest symptom

*254. **Carcinoma of the colon**
- A spreads to epicolic lymph nodes
- B presents as an emergency in 25% of cases
- C is present on the left side in 75% of cases
- D is normally radiosensitive

255. **Which of the following is not a faecal fistula?**
- A Pyelostomy
- B Ileostomy
- C Colostomy
- D Caecostomy

*256. **The complications of colostomy include**
 A prolapse
 B tenesmus
 C stenosis
 D hernia

*257. **Dynamic intestinal obstruction may be due to**
 A paralytic ileus
 B a bolus of food
 C adhesions
 D a gallstone

*258. **The important symptoms of intestinal obstruction include**
 A pain
 B vomiting
 C board-like rigidity
 D constipation

259. **Which is the least important in the treatment of acute obstruction of the small intestine?**
 A A full blood count
 B Gastroduodenal suction
 C Replacement of fluids and electrolytes
 D Operation

260. **Intussusception is not related to**
 A a submucous lipoma
 B swollen Peyer's patches
 C an inverted Meckel's diverticulum
 D a Littre's hernia

*261. **Post-operative paralytic ileus is suspected if there is**
 A colic
 B no passage of flatus
 C no borborygmi
 D effortless vomiting

*262. **In acute appendicitis:**
 A Rigidity may be absent if the appendix is retrocaecal
 B Rigidity may be absent if the appendix is pelvic
 C Vomiting usually precedes pain
 D Classically the pain begins around the umbilicus

*263. **Appendicectomy is indicated for**
  A mucocoele
  B Crohn's disease
  C acute appendicitis
  D diverticula

*264. **A pilonidal sinus occurs**
  A commonly in blondes
  B between the fingers
  C at the umbilicus
  D in the natal cleft

*265. **An anal fissure is**
  A a complication of an anal fistula
  B sometimes due to carcinoma of the anus
  C painful during defaecation
  D a cause of acquired megacolon

*266. **A thrombosed external haemorrhoid is not**
  A painless
  B capable of self-resolution
  C unlike a semi-ripe blackcurrant in appearance
  D best treated by masterly inactivity

*267. **An ischiorectal abscess**
  A may be tuberculous in origin
  B is an infective necrosis of the fat of the ischiorectal fossa
  C requires deroofing
  D should be treated entirely by antibiotics

*268. **Carcinoma of the rectum**
  A is squamous-celled
  B can occur in youth
  C causes bleeding which is slight in amount
  D simulates internal haemorrhoids

*269. **Malignant tumours of the anus**
  A include basaloid tumours
  B primarily spread to the inferior mesenteric lymph nodes
  C may well be treated by radiotherapy
  D simulate anal fissure

*270. Regarding burst abdomen (abdominal dehiscence):
- A   Lower abdominal incisions disrupt more frequently than upper abdominal incisions
- B   It is likely in jaundiced patients
- C   It may present as small bowel obstruction
- D   It is unlikely to recur after suture

*271. The complications of a hernia include
- A   irreducibility
- B   obstruction without strangulation
- C   inflammation
- D   enterocoele

*272. A direct inguinal hernia
- A   is a hernia through the transversalis fascia
- B   may extend into the scrotum
- C   may contain bladder as part of the wall of the sac
- D   has its neck always medial to the inferior epigastric artery

273. Which should not be advised as the treatment of a femoral hernia?
- A   Lockwood's operation
- B   Lotheissen's operation
- C   A truss
- D   McEvedy's operation

*274. A para-umbilical hernia is
- A   congenital
- B   five times more frequent in women than in men
- C   likely to become strangulated if large
- D   treated by the Mayo type of operation

275. A ventral hernia is
- A   femoral
- B   inguinal
- C   obturator
- D   incisional

276. An epigastric hernia is
- A   a Spigelian hernia
- B   a fatty hernia of the linea alba
- C   a type of umbilical hernia
- D   divarication of the rectus abdominis muscles

277. Which of the following is incorrect regarding the diagnosis and management of post-renal anuria?
   A Crystals may be a cause
   B Pain in the loin becoming constant
   C Nephrostomy may be required
   D If no stone is seen on x-ray the kidney on the side which is less painful should be explored

*278. Congenital cystic disease of the kidneys
   A is an hereditary disease transmitted by either parent
   B may be accompanied by similar disease in the pancreas and lung
   C is usually unilateral
   D is commonly complicated by pyelonephritis

279. Which is the least acceptable in the management of a patient with an injury to the kidney?
   A Morphine
   B Bed rest
   C An intravenous urogram
   D Nephrectomy

*280. Hydronephrosis
   A is due to complete obstruction to the outflow of urine from a kidney
   B can be caused by phimosis
   C is related to Dietl's crisis
   D is treated with the overall aim of conserving renal tissue

281. Strangury means
   A the same as tenesmus
   B an intense desire to pass urine
   C the desire to micturate remains unappeased after micturition and painful straining occurs
   D pain on micturition

*282. In chronic pyelonephritis
   A dull lumbar pain is present in some 60% of cases
   B hypertension is present in some 40% of cases
   C casts are found frequently in the urine
   D white cells in the urine may go as high as several million/ml

*283. **A pyonephrosis**
    A is a carbuncle of the kidney
    B is infection of an hydronephrosis
    C is a complication of renal calculus
    D presents as anaemia, fever and loin swelling

284. **A Wilm's tumour is**
    A a retinoblastoma
    B a ganglioneuroma
    C a nephroblastoma
    D a hypernephroma

*285. **The presentation of adenocarcinoma of the kidney includes**
    A women are more often affected than men, the ratio being 2:1
    B polycythaemia
    C clot colic
    D a rapidly developing varicocoele

*286. **The treatment of retention of urine includes**
    A reassurance
    B a hot bath
    C relief by catheterisation and review as an outpatient in 48 hours
    D papaveretum (*e.g.* Omnopon)

*287. **Acquired urinary fistula includes**
    A vesicovaginal
    B vesicocolic
    C ureterovaginal
    D ectopia vesicae

*288. **The clinical features of papilloma of the bladder include**
    A clot retention
    B painless haematuria
    C periodic haematuria
    D pain in the perineum

*289. **Operative urinary diversion is indicated**
    A when the bladder has been removed
    B in case of ectopia vesicae
    C when the bladder sphincters have lost their normal neurological control
    D as a routine in the treatment of vesicovaginal fistula

*290. **Benign enlargement of the prostate**
   A is an involutional hyperplasia
   B affects the submucosal group of glands
   C affects the middle lobe
   D affects the prostatic glands proper

*291. **Individual indications for prostatectomy include**
   A frequency
   B residual urine of 200 ml or more
   C stone
   D venous bleeding

*292. **Metastases from carcinoma of the prostate may be discovered by**
   A the finding of elevated acid phosphatase in the blood
   B x-rays of bone showing osteolytic areas
   C bone scanning
   D scalene node biopsy

*293. **In the treatment of carcinoma of the prostate**
   A radical cure by surgery plays a large part
   B stilboestrol causes improvement in some 85% of cases
   C subcapsular orchiectomy is an alternative to stilboestrol
   D supervoltage x-ray may be used

294. **Which of the following statements is incorrect?**
   A In bladderneck obstruction there is a hypertrophied inter-ureteric bar
   B Spina bifida is the usual cause of retention of urine of neurological origin in childhood
   C Hypospadias is the commonest congenital malformation of the urethra
   D Congenital valves of the posterior urethra obstruct the ingress of a catheter but allow the outflow of urine

295. **Regarding extraperitoneal rupture of the bladder, which statement is incorrect?**
   A Usually there are signs of a fractured pelvis
   B Shock is present
   C The organ will be palpable
   D Catherisation is not permitted

*296. Symptoms of urethral stricture include
- A morning 'dewdrop'
- B dribbling urine after micturition
- C gleet
- D patient has to wait before urine stream begins

297. The following, except one, are related to gonorrhoea in the female:
- A Bartholinitis
- B Vulval warts
- C Ophthalmic neonatorum
- D Ureterocoele

298. Precancerous lesions of the penis exclude
- A leukoplakia of the glans
- B Littritis
- C chronic penile papilloma
- D Paget's disease

299. Regarding incomplete descent of the testis, one of the following statements is incorrect:
- A An indirect or interstitial hernia is present in 70% of cases
- B There is an increased liability to malignant disease
- C Orchiectomy is frequently necessary
- D Atrophy even before puberty may occur

*300. Regarding a hydrocoele:
- A It is almost always translucent
- B One can 'get above the swelling'
- C The testis is separate from the swelling
- D It may obscure an inguinal hernia

PART II
DETERMINATE RESPONSE (YES AND NO) IN SERIES

Note: Continue with the pencil marking × for Yes and − for No as you wish. On an examination computerised form read the instructions carefully as to how to indicate Yes and No. Only Yes answers are printed.

PART II. DETERMINATE

301. In the healing of wounds:
    A   Healing by the first attempt is known as healing by first intention
    B   To suture means to 'bind together'
    C   Skin edges can be approximated by adhesive materials
    D   If the wound has to be sutured for a second time this is called healing by second intention
    E   Healing by second intention usually involves the laying down of more scar tissue

302. The factors which are unfavourable in the healing of a wound of the lower leg include
    A   jaundice
    B   tension
    C   avitaminosis B
    D   diabetes
    E   no haematoma

303. The principles of the closure of wounds include
    A   incised wounds are closed by primary suture
    B   delayed primary suture of a wound only applies to gunshot and missile injuries
    C   skin grafting is not a method of wound closure which can be used as a primary treatment of a wound
    D   the word debridement means to 'unleash' a wound
    E   secondary suture is really the same as delayed primary suture

304. The effects of bullet and bomb injuries include the following principles:
    A   A soft nose bullet travelling at 1200 feet per second causes severe cavitation of a muscle wound with much tissue necrosis
    B   A high velocity bullet passes through the muscle mass of a limb quickly and with comparatively little tissue destruction
    C   The kinetic energy (KE) released by a missile is calculated from the formula $KE = MV$ where M is the mass and V is the velocity
    D   Injury from bombs is also due to the effect of pressure wave of over a thousands pounds per square inch ($6895 kN/m^2$)
    E   Bomb blast has a particularly serious effect on the lungs

305. **The important things to do in the operative surgery of missile injuries is to**
　　A　excise plenty of skin from the wound margin in order to gain access and encourage drainage afterwards
　　B　incise the deep fascia widely
　　C　unite severed nerves
　　D　remove any pieces of bone if part of a comminuted fracture
　　E　pack the wound tightly

306. **Concerning the principle organism of sepsis:**
　　A　The pathogenic *staphylococcus* aureus is coagulase negative
　　B　Group A haemolytic streptococci occur in clusters
　　C　*Escherichia coli* are resistant to penicillin
　　D　*Pseudomonas aeruginosa* causes a blue-green discharge
　　E　*Proteus* in a urinary infection makes the urine acid

307. **Concerning the clinicopathological aspects of sepsis:**
　　A　If antibiotics are used solely as the treatment of an abscess an antibioma may occur
　　B　Cellulitis is usually due to the *staphylococcus albus*
　　C　Erysipelas is an acute dermatitis in secondary syphilis
　　D　Bacteraemia and septicaemia are essentially the same but different in degree
　　E　Disseminated intravascular coagulation is a feature of septicaemia

308. **Regarding tetanus infection:**
　　A　The disease is produced by the endotoxin of *bacillus tetani*
　　B　The toxin travels along nerves to the central nervous system
　　C　The spasms can stop respiration
　　D　A child under the age of one year has an inborn immunity to the disease
　　E　Active immunity is conferred by giving A.T.G. (human anti-tetanus globulin)

309. **In gas gangrene**
　　A　a clostridial myositis occurs
　　B　the patient is flushed, pyrexial and drowsy
　　C　a plain x-ray materially helps in the diagnosis
　　D　if the liver becomes affected it is called a 'foaming liver'
　　E　successful treatment is dependent upon blood transfusion and penicillin

310. **Leprosy**
   A is known as Hansen's disease
   B is caused by a mycobacterium which is acid fast like tuberculosis
   C is spread by direct contact and the fomites
   D if the lepromatous type, causes sharply localised lesions
   E causes deformities due to anaesthesia and misuse which can be treated by a surgeon

311. **Syphilis**
   A is caused by the trepanosome
   B appears as a primary sore 3–4 months after infection
   C is diagnosed in the primary chancre by finding the organisms by dark field microscopy
   D if in the secondary stage is non-infective as it is an immune response and does not feature the spirocheates
   E basically in its pathology causes an endarteritis obliterans

312. **In the causation of skin cancer which of the following are relevant?**
   A The kukri
   B The spinning jenny
   C Chimneys
   D The kangri
   E Asphalt

313. **Carcinoma**
   A spreads by antegrade lymphatic permeation
   B spreads by retrograde lymphatic permeation
   C is a dormant cancer if it is a carcinoma *in situ*
   D can, as a 'kiss cancer', spread from one individual to another by kissing
   E is mesenchymal in origin

314. **Lipomas**
   A are ubiquitous
   B are referred to in general as Dercum's disease
   C tend to occur under anatomical layers of tissue
   D may undergo saponification
   E are not found in the tongue

315. Concerning von Recklinghausen's disease of nerves:
A It is related to osteitis fibrosa cystica
B It is inherited
C It arises in the neurilemmal cells
D If it is plexiform it causes grotesque features
E Sarcomatous changes may occur

316. Cysts
A are always tense on examination
B do not occur in muscle
C can be distinguished from a lipoma on transillumination
D are a feature of filariasis
E may become calcified

317. A fistula will persist if
A a foreign body is present
B a streptococcal infection is present
C tuberculosis is present
D the walls become lined with epithelium
E there is unrelieved obstruction distal to the fistula

318. Concerning the types and features of haemorrhage:
A In arterial haemorrhage the bleeding comes only from the arterial opening nearest the heart
B Venous haemorrhage from a groin wound requires no more treatment than a pressure dressing for four hours
C A 'warning' haemorrhage is characteristic of reactionary haemorrhage
D Secondary haemorrhage is due to a slipped ligature within twelve hours of operation
E A patient with acute blood loss always has a low blood pressure

319. Regarding the measurement of blood loss:
A Blood clot the size of a clenched fist is roughly equal to 500 ml
B Moderate swelling in a fractured shaft of femur may contain as much as 2000 ml of blood
C Total blood and fluid loss during operation is about twice that measured by weighing the swabs in a thoraco-abdominal operation
D Blood volume loss can simply be measured by the haematocrit
E Blood volume can be measured by monitoring the central venous pressure (CVP)

320. **In the management of haemorrhage and shock:**
   A Morphine is a good drug if given intramuscularly
   B Simple pyrexial reactions to blood transfusion are usually due to pyrogens
   C Dextrans are solutions of polysaccharide polymers
   D Vasoconstrictor drugs should only be given early in treatment
   E Bacteraemic shock requires vigorous aggressive treatment including blood transfusion, hydrocortisone and broad spectrum antibiotics

321. **Regarding water balance in the surgical patient:**
   A Endogenous water released during the oxidation of ingested food amounts to 1000–2000 ml in every 24 hours
   B Small amounts of urine highly coloured with a high specific gravity mean poor renal function
   C In pure water depletion the leading sign is oliguria
   D A diuresis must be watched for as it means that enough water has been given
   E Water intoxication is likely when continuous isotonic (5%) dextrose solution is given intravenously

322. **Regarding sodium depletion:**
   A It can be caused by increased secretion of aldosterone
   B It occurs during the first 48 hours after operation
   C It can follow prolonged gastric aspiration combined with unlimited ingestion of water
   D The subcutaneous tissues feel lax
   E The urine contains little or no chloride

323. **Regarding potassium depletion:**
   A After trauma there is increased excretion of potassium for about 3–4 days
   B Villous tumours of the rectum cause hypokalaemia
   C Hypokalaemia follows prolonged gastroduodenal aspiration
   D Muscular spasms are caused by hypolalaemia
   E Intravenous potassium is safe and can be administered freely

324. Regarding surgical post-operative nutrition of patients:
- A All post-operative patients, after gastric surgery, require intravenous alimentation
- B 2000–4000 calories in 2000–4000 ml of fluid can be given daily
- C High concentrations of carbohydrates tend to cause thrombophlebitis
- D Amino acids should not be given at the same time as carbohydrates
- E Elemental diets are suitable for patients with intestinal fistula

325. Concerning warts:
- A The common wart is an example of a tumour caused by a virus
- B A plantar wart is a corn
- C All of them respond readily to applications of salicylic acid in collodion
- D They may be seborrhoeic in origin
- E They may be venereal

326. Lupus vulgaris
- A is a type of collagen disease affecting the face
- B is so called as it marks the patient's face after the manner of a wolf's face
- C spares the mucous membrane of the mouth and nose
- D is a form of tuberculosis of the skin
- E may lead to the formation of epithelioma in the scar tissue

327. A sebaceous cyst
- A is classed, in histology, as an epidermoid cyst
- B only occurs on the face or scalp
- C may, if ulcerated, become a sebaceous horn
- D usually displays a punctum
- E if chronically infected is called a Potts' puffy tumour

328. The molluscum sebaceum
- A is a sebaceous cyst
- B is called Bowen's disease
- C is an epithelioma
- D is a keratoacanthoma
- E may heal spontaneously

329. An angioma
 A is a type of haematoma
 B is a type of hamartoma
 C is a type of ecchymosis
 D is a premalignant condition of the skin
 E develops from ectoderm

330. Premalignant conditions of the skin include
 A Bowen's disease
 B leukoplakia
 C solar keratosis
 D acanthosis nigricans
 E cylindroma

331. A basal cell carcinoma of the skin
 A is called an epithelioma
 B is radiosensitive
 C usually metastasises to the regional lymph nodes
 D may be cystic
 E is known as a Marjolin's ulcer

332. A malignant melanoma
 A only arises in a pre-existing pigmented naevus
 B is unfortunately common before puberty
 C may be surrounded by a halo
 D may be both melanotic and amelanotic
 E spreads by the lymphatics and not by the blood stream

333. The management of a patient with a deep burn of 20% of the body surface includes
 A morphine
 B blood transfusion
 C Dextran
 D haematocrit readings
 E monitoring urine output

334. The treatment of burns includes
 A cold water in first aid
 B exposure
 C the formation of a good scab
 D excision and grafting
 E baths containing a bactericidal substance

335. **Free grafting of skin includes**
   A pinch grafts
   B full thickness grafts
   C Thiersch grafts
   D pedicle grafts
   E cross leg flap

336. **A patient has arterial disease and has intermittent claudication:**
   A If he has rest pain it is felt in the calf muscles
   B The rest pain is relieved by elevation
   C Hot foot baths are beneficial for his cold feet
   D He may have a prolapsed intervertebral disc which is causing the pain on walking
   E He may have diabetes

337. **Regarding aneurysms:**
   A A saccular aneurysm is a false aneurysm
   B An arteriovenous aneurysm is always congenital in origin
   C Expansile pulsation is an extrinsic sign of aneurysm
   D Gangrene is an intrinsic sign of an aneurysm
   E An aneurysm may be mistaken for an abscess

338. **If a girl aged ten has a congenital arteriovenous fistula in the region of the knee joint**
   A the veins are collapsed
   B the leg of the affected side tends to be shorter than that on the unaffected side
   C the cardiac output is decreased
   D ulceration of the leg above the ankle can occur
   E it can be cured by ligation of the feeding artery

339. **An embolus in a limb is recognised by**
   A complete loss of feeling
   B hyperaemia of the affected limb
   C hyperaesthesia of the affected limb
   D the presence of the Brown Sequard syndrome
   E amaurosis fugax

340. **Regarding fat embolism**
   A It is rare
   B It can follow a bone fracture but not a joint arthroplasty
   C The lungs escape due to the fat by-passing them *via* the paravertebral plexus of veins
   D Petechial haemorrhages occur
   E The patient falls into coma

341. **Usual operations for intermittent claudication include**
    A lumbar sympathectomy
    B obturator neurectomy
    C thrombo-endarterectomy
    D reboring by a Fogarty catheter
    E vein by-pass graft

342. **Operations for an obliterated lower abdominal aorta include**
    A endarterectomy
    B vein by-pass graft
    C excision of the aorta
    D femoro-femoral cross over graft
    E aortofemoral Dacron bifurcation graft

343. **A patient who is beginning to suffer from Buerger's disease (thromboangiitis obliterans)**
    A is usually a man aged 40
    B may well be a woman
    C is always an Ashkanazy Jew
    D suffers from polyarteritis nodosa
    E could get gangrene of the bowel

344. **If a man aged 50 suffers from unilateral Raynaud's phenomenon in the hand one should consider as likely causes:**
    A Raynaud's disease
    B Atherosclerosis of the subclavian artery
    C Buerger's disease
    D Cervical rib
    E Subacute bacterial endocarditis

345. **In a lumbar sympathectomy the sympathetic chain in its usual position is likely to be confused with the**
    A ureter
    B psoas minor
    C genitofemoral nerve
    D ilioinguinal nerve
    E lymphatics

346. **The clinical features of a gangrenous hand include**
    A lack of venous return
    B normal capillary response to pressure
    C lack of warmth
    D discoloration due to the disintegration of haemoglobin
    E bare red granulation tissue

347. **The local treatment of gangrene of the foot includes**
    A daily foot baths
    B local heat by a heat pad
    C local cooling by ice
    D minor surgical toilet
    E a sheepskin

348. **Concerning frostbite of the toes and foot:**
    A It is not uncommon in northern city dwellers
    B Blistering, swelling and gangrene are clinical features
    C The foot should be rewarmed with a hot water bottle or heat pad
    D The part should be rubbed with a dry towel
    E An above knee amputation is usually necessary

349. **If a man aged 25 has thrombophlebitis of the long saphenous vein**
    A he can get pylephlebitis
    B he may have varicose veins
    C he may have Buerger's disease
    D he does not need any treatment
    E proximal ligation is required if signs of pus in the vein are evident

350. **The factors which mitigate against post-operative deep vein thrombosis include**
    A living in Singapore
    B reduction of weight
    C graduated compression elastic stockings worn all the time as an inpatient
    D intravenous saline to dilute the blood
    E polycythaemia vera

351. **The leads to a diagnosis of deep vein thrombosis include**
    A elevated temperature
    B induration and tenderness of calf muscles
    C rest pain relieved by hanging the leg out of bed
    D paraesthesia
    E a venogram

352. **What is acceptable in the management of femoral vein thrombosis?**
    A Bed rest and spiral elastic bandages
    B A venogram
    C Thrombectomy
    D Embolectomy
    E A Mobin Udin umbrella inserted into the vein

353. **Regarding axillary vein thrombosis:**
    A It usually occurs spontaneously
    B It is likely to be due to trauma to the subclavian vein between the clavicle, the subclavius muscle and the first rib
    C The forearm and hand feel tense and painful
    D The subclavian vein should be tied immediately
    E A vein by-pass graft should be inserted

354. **If a female patient presents with the recent appearance of varicose veins of the leg one should always**
    A look for a saphena varix
    B perform a rectal examination
    C perform an abdominal examination
    D feel for a Corrigan's pulse
    E think of Milroy's disease as a cause

355. **The treatment of varicose veins includes**
    A the injection of 5 ml of phenol in arachis oil into the veins
    B the injection of ethanolamine oleate 5%
    C taking a female patient off the contraceptive 'Pill' one month before she is going to begin a course of injections
    D ligature of the common femoral vein
    E stripping the superficial femoral vein

356. Bisgaard's treatment of a venous ulcer includes
- A curettage of the ulcer
- B skin grafting of the ulcer
- C elevation of the whole leg
- D a firm elastic bandage
- E active movements to the calf muscles in elevation and on standing

357. Acute lymphangitis
- A is a common feature of mild bacterial infection
- B is usually due to infection with *streptococcus viridans*
- C may by-pass the lymph nodes immediately proximal to the site of infection
- D should be investigated by emergency lymphangiography
- E should be incised without delay and culture swabs taken

358. Lymphangiography of the leg is performed by
- A an injection of sodium diatrizoate (Hypaque) subcutaneously between the toes
- B injecting sodium diatrizoate retrogradely under pressure into a small vein on the dorsum of the foot
- C dissecting lymphatics through an incision on the dorsum of the foot
- D outlining the lymphatics by a subcutaneous injection of the leg above the ankle with patent blue dye
- E the use of an infusion pump

359. Finding the cause of unilateral lymphoedema of the leg includes
- A taking a family history
- B looking for chronic infection in the foot
- C looking for early malignant disease of the testis
- D looking for filariasis
- E performing a Casoni test

360. Tuberculous lymphadenitis
- A does not occur in the aged
- B can be caused by drinking infected milk
- C displays the presence of Reed-Sternberg cells on histological examination
- D as a rule causes discrete rubbery lymph nodes
- E is the originator of scrofulous dermatitis (the King's Evil)

361. **The histological appearance of Hodgkin's disease includes the presence of**
    A Langerhan's cells
    B eosinophils
    C reticulum cells
    D Hassall's corpuscles
    E acanthotic cells

362. **Which of the following procedures are currently helpful in the assessment of lymphadenoma?**
    A Chest x-ray
    B Intravenous urography
    C Laparotomy
    D Tonsillectomy
    E Block dissection of glands of the neck

363. **Simple steps in the diagnosis of a solitary swelling in the left anterior triangle of the neck of a young woman include**
    A examination of the tonsils
    B a white cell count
    C an x-ray of the chest
    D an excision biopsy of the swelling under local anaesthesia
    E incision of the swelling

364. **Steps in the diagnosis of a solitary nonpulsatile swelling in the left supraclavicular fossa include**
    A examination of the thyroid
    B a white cell count
    C an x-ray of the chest
    D an excision biopsy of the swelling
    E needle biopsy

365. **Concerning aspects of an infected finger:**
    A Antibiotics should always be given when a finger becomes red and painful from infection
    B Painful red infection of the finger with lymphangitis should not be incised unless pus is judged clinically to be present
    C Gangrene of the finger is a complication of an infected finger
    D Death is a complication of an infected finger
    E In most cases the infective organism is *streptococcus viridans*

366. Concerning acute paronychia:
   A   It is a subcuticular infection
   B   If pus forms it tends to spread under the nail
   C   Antibiotics do not abort an early infection
   D   Operation using a bloodless field is not necessary
   E   The best treatment is to avulse the whole nail

367. Concerning the surgery of a pulp infection of the finger:
   A   Only when pus is present should the abscess be uncapped
   B   A long incision is necessary in the long axis of the pulp
   C   A collar-stud abscess may be present
   D   A slough must be looked for and carefully excised
   E   The periosteum of the terminal phalanx should be incised

368. If a patient has a web space infection:
   A   There is considerable oedema of the back of the hand
   B   The patient is kept under observation being given a sling and asked to attend the clinic every day
   C   Antibiotics are withheld until pus has formed
   D   The infection fortunately remains localised to that web space
   E   The space is approached surgically through a transverse incision

369. Concerning acute suppurative tenosynovitis:
   A   It is a potentially fatal condition
   B   The organism may be the *streptococcus haemolyticus*
   C   The whole finger is swollen
   D   The finger is flexed
   E   There is exquisite pain on passive extension

370. The principles of the treatment of infections of the hand include
   A   antibiotic therapy
   B   elevation of the affected limb
   C   a plaster of Paris slab or Cramer wire splint may be used
   D   immediate care to retain active movement is essential
   E   bed rest is not indicated

371. **Regarding hand injuries:**
    A   Primary repair of nerves and tendons is always advisable in any type of hand injury
    B   The hand should be exsanguinated for the operation
    C   An untidy wound should be left open to granulate and heal by second intention
    D   Immediately after operation the hand should be nursed flat
    E   Post-operatively early movement is essential to prevent stiffness

372. **Infection of the heel space:**
    A   Is always caused by treading on a thorn or similar object
    B   Always has a collar-stud extension into a deeper plane
    C   Is due mostly to infection of the fat pad of the heel
    D   Can cause oedema of the ankle
    E   If an abscess forms it has to be opened by an incision on the plantar aspect of the heel

373. **In the management of ingrowing toenail:**
    A   The success of conservative measures depends a great deal on the patient's willingness to help himself
    B   The toenail should be cut across convexly
    C   The corners of the nail should be cut back
    D   Avulsion of the whole nail is the most effective method of treatment
    E   Removal of the germinal matrix on the affected side is the surest means of cure

374. **In the management of acute osteomyelitis:**
    A   Three separate venepunctures on the same occasion are made to obtain blood cultures
    B   X-ray changes (*i.e.* lifting of the periosteum) are seen immediately
    C   Antibiotics should not be given until the results of culture and sensitivity are known
    D   Pus, if its presence is suspected clinically, should be drained by operation
    E   Operation is carried out with the limb exsanguinated

375. **Regarding clinicopathological aspects of acute osteomyelitis:**
    A The bone infarct is called a sequestrum
    B Antibiotics will sterilise a sequestrum
    C Ensheathing new bone is called an involucrum
    D If an involucrum should form it has to be removed before cure is possible
    E Discharge through the involucrum is by means of holes known as cloacae

376. **Acute osteomyelitis**
    A can be fatal in children
    B is an haematogenous infection
    C begins in the epiphysis
    D begins under the periosteum
    E causes infarction of bone

377. **The differential diagnosis of acute osteomyelitis includes**
    A acute suppurative arthritis
    B Paget's disease
    C Beriberi
    D Scurvy
    E Haemarthrosis

378. **Chronic osteomyelitis**
    A causes continuous symptoms and signs over a period of months or years
    B on x-ray may reveal a sequestrum
    C on x-ray may reveal a cavity
    D if a Brodie's abscess, reveals a band of sclerosis around a central lucent area on x-ray
    E nowadays is always cured by a long course of antibiotics

379. **The position of ease which joints take up in acute suppurative arthritis includes**
    A shoulder – abducted
    B elbow – extended and supinated
    C hip – flexed, abducted and internally rotated
    D knee – straight
    E ankle – dorsiflexed

380. **The most suitable positions for ankylosis of a joint include**
    A elbow if unilateral – 90° of extension semi-pronated
    B wrist – slightly dorsiflexed
    C hip – 60° of flexion to allow sitting in a chair
    D knee – 30° of flexion to allow sitting in a chair
    E ankle – at a right angle

381. **Acute suppurative arthritis**
    A may be caused by a penetrating wound
    B may be caused by a compound fracture involving a joint
    C may be due to blood-borne infection with the gonococcus
    D causes the joint to be held in the position of ease
    E tends to end with the formation of a fibrous ankylosis

382. **The diagnosis and management of tuberculous arthritis includes**
    A waiting for a positive culture of the tubercle bacillus before treatment is started
    B biopsy of lymph nodes
    C pus is not evacuated
    D arthrotomy
    E arthrodesis

383. **The features of osteo-arthrosis of the hip include**
    A pain which is felt on walking or standing but not in bed at night
    B the joint tends to become stiff in a position of abduction and internal rotation
    C crepitus may be elicited
    D x-ray shows a narrowing of the joint space
    E x-ray may show bone 'cysts' near the joint

384. **Concerning the pathology of rheumatoid arthritis:**
    A The first tissue to be affected is the cartilage
    B Numerous lymphocytes and plasma cells appear in the synovial membrane
    C The capsule becomes contracted
    D A pannus grows upon the articular cartilage
    E Beneath the pannus the bone remains intact

385. The surgery of rheumatoid arthritis includes
- A bone grafting
- B total replacement arthroplasty
- C ankylosis
- D synovectomy
- E capsular reefing

386. The surgery of osteoarthrosis includes such procedures as
- A arthrodesis of the carpometacarpal joint of the thumb
- B arthrodesis of the knee as a primary procedure
- C total replacement arthroplasty of the knee
- D synovectomy of the hip
- E intertrochanteric osteotomy of the femur

387. Tumours of bones and joints include
- A Krukenberg tumour
- B ameloblastoma
- C chordoma
- D synovioma
- E glomus tumour

388. An osteosarcoma
- A tends to occur in the metaphyseal region of a long bone
- B is restricted to persons in the second and third decades
- C does not destroy normal bone but rather grows on the surface
- D spreads to the regional lymph nodes at an early stage
- E should be confirmed by needle biopsy

389. A chondrosarcoma of bone
- A commonly presents as a pathological fracture
- B affects people particularly in the second decade
- C causes an area of bone destruction with ill-defined edges
- D has a matrix which tends to ossify or calcify
- E can occur in the ilium

390. Ewing's tumour of bone
- A is a giant cell tumour
- B is also a secondary deposit from a ganglioneuroma
- C usually occurs in middle age
- D is characterised by subperiostal new bone formation which gives the appearance of sunray spicules
- E can be treated satisfactorily by resection and the insertion of a prosthesis

391. **Concerning the diagnosis of congenital dislocation of the hip at the earliest possible moment in life:**
    A All obstetricians, midwives and general practitioners can be able to diagnose congenital dislocation of the hip at birth
    B The condition is diagnosed at birth by eliciting a 'click' or a 'clunk' from the hip
    C The sign is known as Barlow's or Von Rosen's sign
    D Trendelenberg's sign is positive
    E Shenton's test is positive

392. **Regarding scoliosis of the spine:**
    A The lateral curvature is nearly always associated with a rotational deformity
    B It is usually congenital in origin and is associated with other congenital anomalies in the body
    C Postural scoliosis affects school children and is treated by gymnastics and lessons in deportment
    D The idiopathic type is due to paralysis of special muscles
    E The spine is balanced by secondary curves in the opposite direction above and below

393. **Slipped femoral epiphysis**
    A tends to occur in overweight boys between 10–18 years
    B is fortunately a unilateral condition
    C is a forward and anterior slip
    D may be sudden or slow
    E is confirmed by a lateral x-ray of the hip

394. **Paget's disease**
    A is rare under the age of forty
    B does not affect bones singly (*e.g.* only the clavicle)
    C is painless
    D begins as an osteoblastic proliferation of coarse vascular bone
    E is frequently complicated by osteogenic sarcoma

395. **Rickets causes**
    A frontal bosses
    B enlarged costochondral junctions
    C sabre tibia
    D Clutton's joints
    E triradiate pelvis

396. **A patient with stenosing tenovaginitis**
    A complains of dyspareunia
    B usually has a monilial infection
    C may suffer from trigger finger
    D has thickening of tendon sheaths to the fingers and thumb
    E is likely to have iritis

397. **A Dupuytren's contracture**
    A is a contraction of flexor tendons
    B commonly involves the index and middle fingers
    C can be present in the foot
    D is treated by tendon lengthening procedures
    E may well be seen in people with epilepsy, cirrhosis of the liver or Peyronie's disease

398. **A ganglion**
    A can be painful
    B can be painless
    C may be due to leakage of synovial fluid through the capsule of a joint
    D must be excised under a local anaesthetic
    E often becomes a 'compound palmar ganglion'

399. **Bursitis in origin may be**
    A traumatic
    B pyogenic
    C gonococcal
    D syphilitic
    E tuberculous

400. **The causes of a neuropathic joint include**
    A syringomyelia
    B poliomyelitis
    C diabetes
    D congenital syphilis
    E acquired syphilis

401. **Regarding flat foot:**
    A Spastic flat foot is associated with a spastic diplegia
    B Infants have flat feet
    C Flat feet are always painful
    D Flat feet in children should be treated without delay
    E The problem of pain is related more to the subtalar and midtarsal joints than to the metatarsophalangeal joints

402. **Hallux rigidus**
    A is most common in women
    B is associated with a varus deformity of the first metatarsal
    C is due to synovitis of the interphalangeal joints
    D is osteoarthrosis of the interphalangeal joints
    E can be treated by a metatarsal bar

403. **In the stages of healing of a fracture**
    A the haematoma is invaded by granulation tissue
    B collagen in proteoglycan is deposited by cells derived from capillary endothelium
    C the bone ends are joined by a type of fibrous tissue
    D the fibrous tissue becomes osseous and is known as Haversian bone
    E Haversian bone turns into callus

404. **The management of a fracture includes**
    A reduction
    B immobilisation
    C maintenance of muscle power
    D preservation of joint mobility
    E rehabilitation

405. **In the management of compound fractures the guidelines include:**
    A It is a surgical emergency
    B Treatment aims at sterilising the fracture site
    C A tourniquet should be used if possible to help the surgeon examine the site
    D The wound should be closed at once in order to prevent secondary infection
    E While the skin is healing the fracture cannot be splinted in plaster

406. **Fractures occurring in children differ from those in adults in the following respects. In children**
    A the fractures unite more slowly
    B malunion can be partly corrected by growth
    C joint stiffness is common after immobilisation
    D immobilisation by splinting is the method of choice in treatment
    E involvement of the epiphyseal plate is uncommon as the plate is stronger than the bone

407. Concerning fractures of the waist of the scaphoid:
- A It occurs typically in thin elderly ladies
- B The clinical features suggest a diagnosis of a sprained wrist
- C There is tenderness in the anatomical snuff-box
- D An A-P and a lateral x-ray of the wrist should show the fracture line immediately
- E The fracture is treated in a plaster for two weeks then the plaster is removed and the wrist mobilised

408. In a Colles' fracture the distal fragment is
- A displaced dorsally
- B rotated dorsally
- C displaced medially
- D rotated medially
- E pronated

409. Concerning supracondylar fracture of the humerus in a child:
- A The injury is caused by a fall on the point of the elbow
- B The displacement includes forward displacement of the distal fragment
- C The elbow swells rapidly
- D Ischaemia of the forearm and hand is a distinct possibility
- E After reduction the child may be allowed to go home provided he or she attends the fracture clinic the next day

410. In fracture of the shaft of the humerus:
- A A butterfly fragment may be present
- B The fracture should be reduced under an anaesthetic
- C The arm should be held by plaster abducted to 60° on a traction frame secured to the body
- D Radial palsy is a complication
- E Pseudarthrosis is common

411. If a patient presents with an acromioclavicular dislocation
- A the coraco-clavicular ligament has also ruptured
- B the clavicle is held in place by the clavipectoral fascia
- C reduction is best maintained by a temporary screw through the clavicle to engage in the coracoid process
- D it is acceptable merely to rest the arm in a sling and to mobilise the shoulder when the pain has settled
- E the late sequel of osteoarthrosis can be treated by excision of the outer end of the clavicle

412. **In fractures involving the ankle joint:**
    A   The stability of the tibio-fibular mortice determines the outcome
    B   If the mortice is disrupted it must be reconstructed
    C   In a third degree external rotation injury the talus is free to slide beneath, and possibly fracture, the posterior margin of the tibia
    D   In an inversion (adduction) injury the medial malleolus may be sheared from the tibia
    E   Diastasis of the inferior tibiofibular joint is caused by a vertical compression injury

413. **Fractures of the tibia and fibula**
    A   are often compound
    B   are suitable for treatment by plaster after manipulative reduction in patients under 16 years
    C   cannot be treated by skeletal traction
    D   are most easily and safely treated by internal fixation with an intramedullary nail or plates and screws
    E   can support weight without a plaster after eight weeks of immobilisation

414. **In dislocation of the patella:**
    A   The patella dislocates to the medial side of the knee
    B   The knee becomes locked
    C   The condition is predisposed to by an unusually high lateral femoral condyle
    D   The condition is liable to recur spontaneously
    E   Patellectomy is the most suitable treatment

415. **Intracapsular fractures of the neck of the femur**
    A   always occur in elderly women and men
    B   may be impacted in abduction
    C   when unimpacted are recognised by a shortened leg which lies in external rotation
    D   are invariably operated on
    E   if unimpacted are unlikely to be followed by non-union

416. **If a patient has avascular necrosis of the head of the femur**
    A   the head has firstly been infarcted
    B   the infarct is painful
    C   steroid therapy may be a cause
    D   irradiation is a cause
    E   infarction of bone shows on x-ray by increased radiolucency

417. In posterior dislocation of the hip
  A the leg is flexed
  B the leg is abducted
  C the leg is externally rotated
  D reduction is usually easy
  E about 10% of dislocations are followed by avascular necrosis of the femoral head

418. Malignant growths involving the vault of the skull include
  A osteitis fibrosa cystica
  B osteoclastoma
  C myeloid epulis
  D adamantinoma
  E nephroblastoma

419. Concerning the types of cerebral injury:
  A In concussion the pulse is full and bounding
  B In concussion there is organic structural damage
  C In cerebral contusion there is organic damage to nerve cells and axons
  D In cerebral contusion the muscles are spastic
  E In cerebral laceration damage to the tip of the temporal lobe causes traumatic anosmia

420. Concerning the nursing of unconscious patients:
  A Constant traction on the tongue with a towel clip is necessary
  B The patient must be nursed in a darkened secluded room
  C The patient should be nursed supine
  D Postural drainage in Coleman's position for an hour at a time helps to prevent pneumonia
  E Tracheostomy is contraindicated

421. Regarding extradural haemorrhage:
  A It is due to the dura becoming forcibly detached from the skull at the site of injury
  B A lucid interval between concussion and cerebral compression is always present
  C Constriction of the pupil on the affected side can always be observed in the course of making a diagnosis
  D Coning is unlikely to occur
  E The patient must be operated upon on the next operating list

422. Subdural haemorrhage
- A is six times less common than extradural haemorrhage
- B is particularly common in young people
- C causes slowing of cerebration which comes and goes
- D may cause a mid-brain pressure cone and a rise of the operative mortality from nil to 30%
- E is characterised by papilloedema

423. Regarding the management of scalp and skull injuries:
- A On examination of the wound in the accident receiving room a finger should be inserted to detect the presence of a compound fracture and brain damage
- B For a closed depressed fracture immediate operation is indicated
- C All scalp wounds should be explored adequately
- D A general anaesthetic is always necessary
- E Any loose pieces of fractured skull should be removed and discarded as they will encourage infection

424. In a patient with an anterior fossa fracture:
- A Proptosis may occur
- B Any subconjunctival haemorrhage is wedge-shaped with the apex at the back
- C The injury usually includes a tear of the tentorium
- D An aerocoele may form
- E The optic nerve is frequently torn

425. The late effects of a head injury include
- A symptomatic fits in the first 24 hours which recur after bruising has subsided
- B post-traumatic hydrocephalus
- C headache which is not cerebral but is spinal in origin
- D Jacksonian epilepsy
- E idiopathic epileptic fits

426. Regarding the diagnosis of intracerebral abscess:
- A General features are more important than focal signs
- B Persistent pyrexia is an important feature
- C As the abscess enlarges the pulse rate may become slower
- D Leucocytosis does not occur because of the blood brain barrier
- E A lumbar puncture should not be performed as it will cause coning

427. The types of glioma of the brain include
- A medulloblastoma
- B acoustic neuroma
- C astrocytoma
- D meningioma
- E oligodendroglioma

428. In cone formation
- A the temporal lobe may be forced downwards into the tentorial opening
- B the cerebellar vermis may be pushed upwards into the tentorial opening
- C the cerebellar tonsils may be forced downwards into the foramen magnum
- D unilateral pupillary dilation is an urgent sign
- E lumbar puncture to drain CSF relieves the condition

429. Regarding the presentation and diagnosis of cerebral tumour:
- A Neurological examination usually indicates the type of tumour
- B A high E.S.R. is strongly suggestive of secondary tumour
- C Primary cerebral tumour is more common than metastatic carcinoma
- D 30% of bronchial carcinomas present with cerebral symptoms before any chest symptoms have occurred
- E Erosion of the posterior clinoid processes suggests that removal of the tumour may be possible

430. Tumours of the pituitary body include those which are
- A basophil
- B acidophil
- C chromophobe
- D craniopharyngiomas
- E neurofibromas

431. In the treatment of hydrocephalus
- A a tumour, if the cause of the obstruction, is removed if possible
- B intracranial shunts may be used for obstruction of the aqueduct of Sylvius
- C a ventricular shunt into the pleural cavity makes use of the Holter valve
- D a ventriculoatrial shunt does not require the use of a valve
- E a ventriculoatrial shunt tube is introduced *via* the common facial vein

432. Regarding subarachnoid haemorrhage:
- A Berry aneurysms are responsible for at least half of the cases
- B The aneurysms are due to atherosclerosis
- C The aneurysms are due to syphilis in 20% of cases
- D No age is exempt
- E 20% of patients have more than one aneurysm

433. In a patient with spinal concussion:
- A A spastic paralysis occurs below the site of the lesion
- B There is abolition of reflex activity below the lesion
- C Joint position sense is lost
- D Pain and temperature sense is lost
- E If there is no partial or complete cord injury power and sensation should take 7–10 days to return

434. The cause of death after a traumatic transection of the cord includes
- A cerebral abscess
- B aerocoele
- C pyelonephritis
- D bedsores
- E surgical emphysema

435. In a fifth cervical complete cord lesion the following are paralysed
- A the arms
- B the chest
- C the diaphragm
- D the legs
- E the platysma

436. Spina bifida may
- A present with foot drop
- B present with enuresis
- C be completely occult
- D be indicated by a hairy patch
- E present as a meningocoele

437. Intramedullary tumours of the cord cause
- A early root pain
- B dissociated sensory loss
- C late bladder symptoms
- D late upper motor neurone paralysis
- E a wide belt of local sensory loss

438. Trigeminal neuralgia
- A is known as tic doloureux
- B is pain mainly in the first division of the fifth nerve
- C is helped by rubbing the part of the face affected
- D is a constant pain
- E is not accompanied by any physical signs

439. Neurapraxia is
- A intrathecal rupture of the nerve fibres within an intact sheath
- B partial or complete division of nerve sheath and fibres
- C physiological paralysis of the intact nerve fibres
- D followed by degeneration of axons
- E followed by complete recovery

440. In recovery from axonotmesis
- A Wallerian degeneration has occurred in the distal portion of the broken axons leaving an empty tubule
- B the Nissl granules reform
- C the proliferating axons grow through the block caused by intraneural fibrosis
- D the downgrowing axons proceed immediately at the rate of 2 mm/day
- E on arrival at the end-organs there is a delay of about three weeks before these end-organs are activated

441. An upper brachial plexus lesion (Erb-Duchenne)
   A   only affects infants after a difficult labour
   B   affects the fifth dorsal nerve root
   C   causes the arm to hang by the side with the forearm pronated
   D   involving the fifth nerve gives rise to an area of anaesthesia over the outer side of the arm
   E   may be treated by ankylosis

442. Severance of the long nerve of Bell (the external respiratory nerve) causes
   A   paralysis of the serratus anterior
   B   paralysis of the subscapularis
   C   winging of the scapula
   D   deficiency of the 'lunge' as in boxing or fencing
   E   difficulty in raising the arm above a right angle from a position in front of the body

443. Severance of the median nerve at the elbow causes
   A   paralysis of all the flexors of the fingers
   B   fixed flexion of the terminal phalanx of the thumb
   C   wasting of the hypothenar muscles
   D   trophic changes in the index finger
   E   loss of sensation at first over the thumb and radial two and a half fingers

444. Severance of the ulnar nerve at the wrist causes
   A   loss of sensation on the anterior and posterior aspects of the inner one and a half fingers
   B   inability to flex the terminal phalanx of the little finger
   C   flexion of the little finger at the metacarpophalangeal joint
   D   inability to abduct or adduct the fingers
   E   a positive Froment's sign

445. Complete severance of the lateral popliteal nerve
   A   may be due to an injury to the upper end of the fibula
   B   may be due to an operation for multiple ligation of varicose veins
   C   causes a talipes equinovarus
   D   causes anaesthesia of the outer sides of the 4th and 5th toes
   E   causes anaesthesia of the front of the ligamentum patellae

446. The causes of proptosis include
   A   arteriovenous fistula (cavernous sinus/internal carotid artery)
   B   a cavernous sinus thrombosis
   C   haemorrhage into the orbit
   D   orbital cellulitis
   E   leukaemia

447. A retinoblastoma
   A   is a type of ganglioneuroma
   B   is a malignant undifferentiated tumour
   C   may be hereditary
   D   is locally invasive and does not cause metastases
   E   can be treated by radiotherapy

448. In the differential diagnosis and management of the 'acute red eye':
   A   A drop of fluorescein will show up corneal ulceration
   B   Conjunctivitis does not affect vision
   C   Steroid drops are used for keratitis
   D   In glaucoma there is an exudate in the anterior chamber and the pupil is notched
   E   The vomiting in glaucoma may be mistaken as a symptom of an acute abdominal emergency

449. In the treatment of cleft lip and cleft palate
   A   Both should be repaired at the age of two years
   B   In repair of the cleft lip the object is to obtain closure without shortening the upper lip
   C   In repair of the cleft palate the object is to achieve adequate speech and dentition
   D   In cleft palate the repair means suturing both nasal and pharyngeal layers after suitable tension releasing procedures
   E   If the premaxilla is unfused and juts out it has to be excised before repair can be carried out.

450. A preauricular sinus
   A   is a type of pilonidal sinus
   B   may be bilateral
   C   is found on the root of the helix or on the tragus
   D   is cured by incision and being allowed to heal from the deeper layers
   E   may be mistaken for a tuberculous sinus

451. **In a motor accident a young woman has been thrown forward through the windscreen as she has not been wearing a seat belt:**
    A The immediate danger is blood loss
    B The patient is transported supine in the ambulance
    C There is usually a lot of blood to be seen and this accounts for the shock
    D Excision of dead tissue is reduced to a minimum
    E Suture of the skin alone will suffice

452. **One of the types of fracture of the maxilla is suggested by**
    A the type of accident
    B fish face deformity
    C open bite deformity
    D diplopia
    E CSF otorrhoea

453. **Dental caries increases the risk of morbidity from surgical procedures. It favours the occurrence of**
    A stomatitis
    B parotitis
    C bacteriaemia
    D lung abscess
    E acute pyelonephritis

454. **The common and important epithelial odontomes are the**
    A dental cyst
    B myeloid epulis
    C dentigerous cyst
    D adamantinoma
    E giant-celled reparative granuloma

455. **The clinical features of carcinoma of the maxillary antrum include**
    A toothache
    B free bleeding on proof puncture of the antrum
    C epiphora
    D entropion
    E proptosis

456. Epistaxis
- A is commonly epistaxis digitorum
- B usually comes from veins in Little's area
- C is a feature of hypertension
- D if coming from the front of the nose the treatment is to pack the nostrils
- E sometimes requires arterial ligation

457. Otitis externa
- A is also known as telephonist's ear
- B is usually caused by trauma to and infection of a sebaceous cyst
- C can be caused by seborrhoea
- D is treated by being syringed daily
- E requires that the feet be inspected and treated if relevant

458. Carcinoma of the pinna
- A is an extension of carcinoma of the auditory canal
- B is known as Singapore ear
- C is a basal-celled carcinoma
- D is best treated by radiotherapy
- E may require the ear to be cut off

459. A patient with serous otitis media
- A is usually a young man or woman
- B may have an allergy which blocks the Eustachian tube
- C is said to have 'glue ear'
- D has a bulging red ear drum
- E may require the insertion of a grommet

460. Concerning aspects of stomatitis:
- A It can be caused by any injury to the mouth
- B Aphthous stomatitis means stomatitis caused by fungal infection
- C It is favoured by malnutrition
- D Foot and mouth disease affects cattle, not man
- E It is a feature of Vincent's angina

461. Leukoplakia is
- A another name for chronic superficial glossitis
- B a slowly progressive hyperkeratosis
- C recognised in the early stages as a thin milky film
- D restricted to the mouth and tongue
- E not a premalignant condition

462. Regarding ulcers of the tongue:
 A Recurrent aphthous ulcers are contagious so kissing is to be avoided
 B A tuberculous ulcer is painless
 C A dental ulcer caused by a sharp tooth can be diagnosed with confidence
 D A Wasserman reaction can be a hindrance rather than a help
 E A negative biopsy clears the patient of having a cancer of the tongue

463. If a patient has a carcinoma of the tongue:
 A The patient is most likely to be an old man
 B The patient may well be a woman aged 40
 C Attention is drawn to it early on by the appearance of blood-stained salivation
 D Pain may be felt in the ear
 E The overall five-year survival rate after treatment is about 25%

464. In the palliative treatment of carcinoma of the tongue
 A radiotherapy has no value
 B surgical resection of a recurrence may be feasible
 C cryosurgery is useful
 D pain may be relieved by blocking the fifth nerve
 E morphine should be avoided as it depresses respiration

465. Regarding the anatomy of the salivary glands:
 A The parotid gland lies deep to the branches of the facial nerve
 B The socia parotidis lies below and behind the ear over the mastoid process
 C The parotid duct opens in the mouth opposite the upper canine tooth
 D The submandibular gland lies in the submental triangle
 E The submandibular gland empties by several small ducts into the floor of the mouth

466. Acute parotitis
 A may be due to nonspecific bacterial infection
 B may be due to the Coxsachie A virus
 C is likely in the post-operative period following major surgery
 D requires immediate incision
 E with pus formation is recognised straightaway by fluctuation

467. Concerning salivary calculi:
- A Submandibular stones in the duct are removed *via* the floor of the mouth
- B Submandibular stones in the gland are extracted from the gland through an incision in the neck
- C Parotid calculi are more common than submandibular calculi
- D Salivary stones contain calcium carbonate
- E A parotid duct stone causes cysts of the parotid

468. In the management of a pleomorphic adenoma of the parotid
- A a biopsy is taken
- B operation is advised
- C the tumour is enucleated
- D partial parotidectomy with conservation of the facial nerve is preferred
- E post-operative radiotherapy is given

469. A branchial cyst
- A commonly appears between the 20th and 25th years
- B arises from the vestigial remnants of the fourth branchial cleft
- C is usually lined by squamous epithelium
- D does not become inflamed like neighbouring lymph nodes
- E may be contiguous with a track which passes through the fork of the carotid artery as far as the pharyngeal wall

470. Regarding a cervical rib:
- A It can always be felt in the neck
- B The bone of the rib is always the cause of the symptoms
- C It can cause ischaemic muscle pain in the forearm
- D Trophic changes can occur in the fingers
- E Treatment is subperiosteal excision of the rib

471. In tuberculous lymphadenitis of the neck
- A the patient may be an elderly lady
- B the bovine bacillus is mostly responsible
- C a primary focus in the lungs may be present
- D the nodes tend to be matted together
- E a collar-stud abscess may form

472. Regarding a carotid body tumour:
  A The tumour is pulsatile
  B It is easy to dissect from the carotid artery
  C At operation it may well be necessary to use a temporary by-pass while a vein graft is being inserted
  D If the internal carotid artery is simply ligated in the removal of the tumour death or hemiplegia follows in 33% of cases
  E Recurrence is unusual after complete resection

473. The blood vessels to and from the thyroid including name and branch or tributary are:
  A The superior thyroid artery, being a branch of the internal carotid artery
  B The middle thyroid vein – a tributary of the external jugular vein
  C The middle thyroid artery – a branch of the external carotid artery
  D The inferior thyroid artery – a branch of the thyrocervical trunk
  E The inferior thyroid veins – tributaries of the innominate veins

474. Myxoedema
  A is an advanced form of juvenile hypothyroidism
  B is related to thyroidectomy and ^{131}I therapy
  C is a cause of carpal tunnel syndrome
  D returns a serum T^4 below 3·0 µg/100 ml (60 mmol/l)
  E is treated by d-thyroxine

475. Regarding simple goitre:
  A It may be sporadic which means that it is prevalent in a people or a district
  B A diffuse hyperplastic goitre feels firm to hard on palpation
  C A nodular goitre tends to be painful
  D A nodular goitre may be complicated by a follicular carcinoma
  E All types of simple goitre are more common in the female than in the male

476. Concerning the clinicopathological features of hyperthyroidism:
A It may occur at any age
B Enophthalmos is a characteristic feature
C Cardiac arrhythmias are superimposed on the sinus tachycardia
D Myaesthenia gravis is a late feature
E Histology reveals acini lined by flattened cuboidal epithelium filled with homogenous colloid

477. Exophthalmos
A is a proptosis of the eye
B is due to retrobulbar infiltration with fluid and round cells
C associated upper eyelid spasm and retraction may be improved by B-adrenergic drugs as eye drops
D can be complicated by chemosis
E can proceed to a malignant variety which causes secondary deposits in the liver ('beware the glass eye and the large liver')

478. Regarding antithyroid drugs in the treatment of thyrotoxicosis:
A Thiouracil is commonly used
B Propyl thiouracil has been given up
C Iodides are sound in the long term
D Potassium perchlorate is infrequently used
E Carbimazole is in common use

479. The steps in the operation of subtotal thyroidectomy include
A general anaesthesia by an endotracheal tube
B an H-shaped incision
C dividing the middle thyroid artery
D identification of the course of the recurrent laryngeal nerves
E haemostasis by diathermy of veins leaving the thyroid

480. In patients with medullary carcinoma of the thyroid:
A Other members of the family may be affected
B Constipation is a feature in 30% of cases
C A phaeochromocytoma may be present
D Neuromas can occur on the tongue
E The tumour is hormone dependant

481. A lingual thyroid
- A forms a swelling in the upper part of the neck
- B is associated with struma ovarii – part of an ectopic ovarian teratoma
- C can be excised without any difficulty or hormonal problem
- D is likely to shrink if the patient is given L-thyroxine
- E is related to the foramen caecum

482. Regarding the parathyroid glands:
- A 5% are found in the upper mediastinum
- B The 'chief' cells produce parathormone
- C Parathormone stimulates osteoblastic activity
- D Parathormone reduces the renal tubular reabsorbtion of phosphate
- E Calcitonin is secreted by the oxyphil cells of the parathyroid

483. Regarding parathyroid tetany:
- A It is a common complication of subtotal thyroidectomy
- B The symptoms appear immediately on recovery from the anaesthetic
- C Acrocyanosis occurs
- D Symptoms can be relieved by 10–20 ml of 10% solution of calcium gluconate
- E The level of serum calcium should be estimated daily as a guide to calcium dosage

484. The clinical features of hyperparathyroidism are concerned with
- A bones
- B stones
- C abdominal groans
- D psychic moans
- E retinal cones

485. Radiography is useful in the delineation of an adrenal tumour because
- A urography shows a deformity of the upper calyx of the kidney
- B paracoccygeal injection of oxygen is a good way of showing up the tumour when the oxygen reaches the upper retroperitoneal area
- C selective arteriography will show a vascular blush
- D calcification in an adrenal is characteristic
- E the twelfth rib is eroded

486. The adrenal cortex
A contains the glomerular zone
B contains the acanthotic layer
C contains the reticular zone
D makes androgens
E is inhibited by ACTH

487. Types of hypercorticism include
A Conn's syndrome
B Simmond's disease
C Addison's disease
D Cushing's syndrome
E Adrenogenital syndrome

488. In a child with a neuroblastoma of the adrenal
A the disease begins in the cortex
B the age of the child is most likely to be over seven years
C a left-sided primary tends to give rise to secondaries in the orbit and skull
D a right-sided primary tends to give rise to large liver metastases
E spontaneous remission is known to occur

489. Retraction of the nipple
A is always unilateral
B in men is due to wearing braces
C is an important factor in the cause of breast abscess
D if recent can be due to a chancre
E can be caused by fat necrosis

490. A breast abscess
A may follow mumps
B first goes through a stage of milk engorgement
C goes through a stage of bacterial mastitis
D is usually caused by the haemolytic streptococcus
E should be treated with a broad spectrum antibiotic

491. In a patient with fibroadenosis of the breast
A duct papillomatosis may be present
B pregnancy usually produces relief
C the breasts feel nodular and the periphery has a saucer-like edge
D radiotherapy is a useful palliative treatment
E the breasts should be replaced by prosthetic implants

492. **Regarding duct papilloma of the breast:**
    A It commonly occurs in women between 35 and 50 years
    B A cystic swelling may be felt beneath the areola
    C Multiple papillomas are most unusual
    D Local mastectomy is usually indicated
    E Microdochectomy is a suitable operation

493. **Regarding carcinoma of the breast:**
    A The malignant cells transgress the internal elastic lamina of a duct
    B The medullary (anaplastic) type feels stony hard
    C The atrophic scirrhous type occurs in younger women
    D *Peau d'orange* of the skin is an early sign of carcinoma
    E It is virtually impossible clinically to distinguish a duct papilloma from a duct carcinoma

494. **In the generally accepted clinical staging of carcinoma of the breast**
    A in Stage I an area of adherence to the skin smaller than the periphery of the tumour does not affect staging
    B in Stage II axillary nodes are palpable and immobile
    C the absence of palpable nodes means that carcinoma has not spread to them
    D if the tumour is fixed to the pectoral muscle but not to the chest wall it is nevertheless Stage IV
    E cancer *en cuirasse* is included in Stage IV

495. **In the endocrine treatment of carcinoma of the breast**
    A 15% of patients can be cured by giving hormones
    B oophorectomy is only of value after the menopause
    C androgens are contraindicated
    D oestrogens should not be given unless the woman is over 40 years
    E adrenalectomy is best carried out through a Pfannenstiel's incision

496. **If a patient has a quinsy**
    A his or her age is usually between 8–18 years
    B it is a retropharyngeal abscess
    C saliva dribbles from the mouth
    D the uvula is displaced
    E a general anaesthetic is essential

497. Angiofibroma of the nasopharynx
- A is a benign tumour
- B never metastasises
- C is highly destructive
- D causes a 'frog face'
- E occurs in boys

498. Cryosurgery can be used for
- A palliation of painful uncontrolled cancers
- B prostatic enlargement
- C piles
- D Paget's disease of the nipple
- E perniosis

499. If a child suddenly has an impacted foreign body in the larynx
- A it may be dislodged by inverting the child and slapping its back
- B a finger should not be used to try and dislodge and hook out the object
- C immediate tracheostomy is not called for
- D the child should be sent to an E.N.T. surgeon
- E cardiac arrest is unlikely to occur

500. Regarding acute oedema of the glottis:
- A It is oedema of the vocal cords
- B Some cases are due to angioneurotic oedema
- C Dysphagia may be present
- D If observed through the laryngoscope it looks like the cervix
- E Morphine is used to allay stridor

501. If the chest is crushed in a motor accident
- A the aorta can be ruptured
- B paradoxical movement is likely to occur
- C early treatment is directed at improving ventilation
- D morphine should not be given
- E tracheostomy is best delayed until repeated bronchoscopy is insufficient to remove tracheobronchial secretions

502. **An empyema**
    A   is a pleural abscess
    B   is often primary
    C   may contain staphylococci
    D   may require decortication
    E   is best drained by open rib resection as soon as the diagnosis is made

503. **Carcinoma of the bronchus**
    A   usually presents with haemoptysis
    B   should be suspected if an attack of 'influenza' does not resolve
    C   does not occur in non-smokers
    D   secondary deposits and finger clubbing frequently go together
    E   carries a prognosis of a 20% five-year cure rate after radical resection

504. **Amongst the clinical features and management of pulmonary oedema is included**
    A   thin frothy haemoptysis
    B   x-ray of the chest shows a bat wing appearance
    C   morphine given intravenously is particularly effective in left ventricular failure
    D   Aminophylline should be given as 250 mg i.v. rapidly
    E   positive pressure ventilation is effective

505. **Regarding pulmonary embolism:**
    A   Small emboli may be silent
    B   Multiple small emboli can cause pulmonary hypertension
    C   Medium emboli cause atelectasis of a segment or lobe
    D   With a large embolus an E.C.G. may show left ventricular strain
    E   A massive pulmonary embolus causes death through atrial fibrillation

506. **When extracorporeal circulation is used in open cardiac surgery**
    A   blood is withdrawn from one femoral artery, oxygenated and pumped into the left atrium
    B   the blood is diverted from the heart and lungs
    C   the time limit is one hour
    D   the patient has to be cooled to 29–30°C
    E   a ventricular septal defect can be repaired

507. The clinical features of coarctation of the aorta include
- A headaches
- B well developed shoulders compared with the pelvis
- C Corrigan's pulse
- D intermittent claudication
- E warm vasodilated extremities

508. Artificial pacemakers
- A can be wholly external using electrodes applied to the surface of the chest
- B can be wholly internal, battery-operated, which is buried in the abdominal wall
- C can be combined internal and external
- D are designed to work for one year
- E act *via* catheter electrodes passed retrogradely in an artery into the left ventricle

509. Regarding perforation of the oesophagus:
- A It can occur below an oesophageal stricture when a bougie is passed
- B A plain x-ray is better than a barium swallow for diagnosis
- C An oesophagoscopy should be performed to observe the position and extent of the tear
- D The patient should be treated conservatively if an immediate diagnosis is made
- E Patients with delayed symptoms and negative x-rays are treated by massive antibiotic therapy and parenteral feeding

510. The indication for operation on an hiatus hernia include
- A attributable refractile anaemia
- B the presence of a duodenal ulcer
- C inability to lose weight
- D stenosis
- E gastro-oesophageal reflux

511. The Plummer-Vinson syndrome
- A was described earlier by Paterson and Kelly
- B nearly always affects a middle-aged man
- C includes retching and choking symptoms as characteristic
- D includes the formation of webs
- E is not premalignant

512. Regarding miscellaneous lesions of the oesophagus:
  A Scleroderma of the oesophagus is a variety of Crohn's disease
  B A Schatzki's ring is a metal button used for anastomosing the oesophagus after resection
  C A lye stricture is a pseudostricture
  D A leiomyoma can occur in the oesophagus
  E Presbyoesophagus is corkscrew oesophagus

513. Gastric mucus
  A is produced by the parietal cells
  B has a pH of 5·2 to 6·8
  C has considerable buffering capacity
  D protects the alkaline gastric mucosa
  E is composed of glycoprotein

514. In general the symptoms of a duodenal ulcer include
  A pain soon after eating but not when lying down
  B considerable vomiting
  C afraid to eat
  D heartburn
  E night pain

515. In a patient with a perforated peptic ulcer:
  A If it is a gastric ulcer it could well be malignant
  B Morphine or other analgesics must not be given until written permission for operation has been obtained
  C It is best to perform a gastroscopy before deciding to operate
  D A perforated duodenal ulcer looks oedematous and punched out
  E It is necessary to drain the subhepatic space and the pelvis

516. A patient admitted and treated conservatively for haematemesis
  A is allowed up to go to the toilet
  B is given morphine 15 mg regularly
  C is given a rapid blood transfusion
  D is allowed nothing by mouth
  E should be given a small enema to see if he has melaena

517. The complications of a duodenal ulcer include
  A pyloric stenosis
  B penetration
  C carcinoma
  D hourglass stomach
  E leather bottle stomach

518. **Specific complications of gastric operations include**
    A duodenal fistula
    B pancreatitis
    C gastrocolic fistula
    D gallstones
    E polycythaemia

519. **If a patient has had a vagotomy for a duodenal ulcer**
    A he is often troubled by obstinate constipation
    B he tends to get 'blown up' with wind
    C a gastric ulcer may occur
    D he tends to suffer from calcium deficiency
    E is very likely to suffer from a bolus obstruction

520. **If a patient has a partial gastrectomy**
    A diarrhoea is common, episodic and troublesome
    B previous tuberculous disease may be reactivated
    C carcinoma of the stomach may occur in the gastric remnant
    D bilious vomiting is intermittent rather than with every meal
    E megaloblastic anaemia is common and appears about a year after the operation

521. **Regarding foreign bodies in the stomach:**
    A If a patient has several foreign bodies in the stomach it is likely that these have been swallowed on purpose
    B They should always be removed promptly by operation
    C They tend to be radiolucent
    D Fibreoptic gastroscopy should replace operations for their removal
    E If they pass round into the jejunum it is likely that they will impact in the ileum

522. **In the haemolytic anaemias**
    A spherocytosis is due to abnormal immunological responses
    B chronic ulcers of the legs occur in congenital haemolytic anaemia
    C the liver may be palpable
    D the patients tend to suffer from gallstones
    E ACTH is the general mainspring of treatment

523. **Purpura may present in a patient who has**
    A ecchymoses
    B portwine staining
    C venous gangrene
    D phlegmasia caerulea dolens
    E acute intestinal obstruction

524. **'Egyptian' splenomegaly**
    A follows amoebic dysentry
    B can be caused by malaria
    C is mostly caused by *Schistosoma haematobium*
    D causes diffuse periportal fibrosis of the liver
    E is often benefitted by splenectomy

525. **Liver function tests in common usage include**
    A secretin-pancreozymin test
    B serum acid phosphatase
    C serum aminotransferases
    D phenolphthalein test
    E serum albumin level

526. **Regarding the anatomy of the liver:**
    A The true boundary between the right and left lobes of the liver is marked by the attachment of the falciform ligament
    B The true boundary between the right and left lobes of the liver is marked by the gall bladder bed
    C The blood from the liver is drained by three major hepatic veins
    D The bile ducts and branches of the portal vein follow the hepatic arterial branches
    E There are no lymphatic vessels in the liver

527. **Regarding chronic abscesses of the liver:**
    A There are many causes but in half the cases no cause can be discovered
    B The presence of leucocytosis is helpful in making the diagnosis
    C Ultrasonic and CT scanning will localise the abscess
    D The condition is fatal unless it is located by laparotomy and drained
    E If the abscess is drained by a drainage tube and it is an amoebic abscess a fatal spreading infection of the abdominal wall called amoebiasis cutis can occur

528. Regarding hydatid disease:
A It is due to a small worm *demodex folliculorum* which enters the body through the pores of the skin
B Dogs are the chief originators of the worm ova
C The worm contains a head with a terminal sucker and a body comprised of one germinal segment
D An ovum is four times the size of a red blood corpuscle and bears two hooklets
E It is unknown in the United Kingdom

529. The causes of cirrhosis of the liver include
A the *entamoeba histolytica*
B ulcerative colitis
C malaria
D schistosmiasis
E nutritional deficiency

530. Suitable methods employed to control bleeding from oesophageal varices include
A splenectomy
B pituitrin
C a Sengstaken tube
D a Fogarty catheter
E injection

531. Regarding radiological investigations of the biliary tree:
A Plain x-ray shows up radiolucent gallstones
B A cholecystogram is performed after breakfast twelve hours following the ingestion of the contrast medium
C Cholecystography is valueless if the plasma bilirubin level is over 3 mg/100 ml (51 μmol/l)
D The contrast medium contains iodine with an atomic weight of 131
E Peroperative cholangiography is desirable in all cholecystectomy operations.

532. Regarding congenital atresia of the bile ducts:
A It tends to be caused by neonatal hepatitis
B Meconium is clay-coloured at birth
C The mother has hereditary spherocytosis
D Operative cholangiography is impossible because of the size of the ducts
E Surgery has very little to offer in such cases

533. Gallstones
- A are always the cause of flatulent dyspepsia
- B are becoming common in post-partum primipara who were pre-pregnancy 'Pill' takers
- C may be present in the newborn
- D cause mucocoele of the gall bladder
- E are present in the common bile duct in 40% of patients with stones in the gall bladder

534. The conservative treatment for acute cholecystitis
- A is avoided in typhoidal cholecystitis
- B has a higher morbidity than emergency operation
- C has a higher mortality than emergency operation
- D only results in resolution in 40% of the cases
- E is likely to reduce the chances of damage to the common bile ducts at an elective operation compared with an emergency operation

535. Cholecystostomy
- A is essentially part of the operation of cholecystectomy
- B should be performed with choledochotomy
- C is reserved for empyema of the gall bladder
- D is performed in a very ill patient instead of cholecystectomy
- E should always be followed by cholecystectomy

536. In at least 15% of patients on whom cholecystectomy has been performed the symptoms for which the operation was performed persist. These could be due to the presence of
- A an abscess of the cystic duct remnant
- B an hiatus hernia
- C a motility disorder of the duodenum and choledochal sphincter
- D pancreatitis
- E a stone remaining in the common bile duct

537. Charcot's biliary triad includes
- A itching of the skin
- B fluctuating jaundice
- C recurrent pain
- D pale stools
- E intermittent fever and rigors

538. Carcinoma of the gall bladder
A is either an extension of carcinoma of the pancreas or a cholangiocarcinoma
B usually starts in the cystic duct and neck of the gall bladder
C may be a squamous cell carcinoma
D is more common in women than in men
E carries a dismal prognosis

539. Mucoviscidosis (fibrocytic disease) of the pancreas
A accompanies congenital cystic disease of the kidneys and liver
B is a manifestation of a hereditary congenital abnormality of mucus secretion
C causes intestinal obstruction
D encourages staphylococcal infections
E causes excessive loss of sodium chloride in the sweat

540. The clinicopathological features of acute pancreatitis may include
A fat necroses
B cholelithiasis
C mumps
D leucopaenia
E sulphaemoglobinaemia

541. If a patient has chronic pancreatitis
A the volume of secretion as a result of the secretinpancreozymin test is reduced
B a needle biopsy to distinguish between it and carcinoma should be performed through the epigastrium should be performed
C alcohol in small quantities is permitted
D an pain is severe, chemical splanchnicectomy under x-ray television control is applicable
E cholecystojejunostomy with enteroenterostomy is suitable if jaundice is present

542. A patient with an insulinoma
A has an alpha-cell tumour of the pancreas
B may be in a mental hospital
C displays Saint's triad and this establishes the diagnosis
D has an identifiable hypoglycaemia with fasting up to 72 hours
E is likely to have the Zollinger-Ellison syndrome

543. The presence of carcinoma of the pancreas can be indicated by
    A thrombophlebitis migrans
    B diabetes
    C pancreatic calcinosis
    D the ordinary 3 sign on a barium meal
    E the triple response of Lewis

544. The subphrenic spaces where abscesses occur are
    A midline extraperitoneal
    B midline intraperitoneal
    C right posterior intraperitoneal
    D in the lesser sac
    E left anterior intraperitoneal

545. Which of the following are forms of peritonitis?
    A Bile
    B Meconium
    C Pneumococcal
    D Streptococcal
    E Starch

546. Regarding paracentesis abdominis:
    A It may be employed in congestive cardiac failure
    B It may be employed for the Arnold-Chiari malformation
    C A local anaesthetic is unnecessary
    D The fluid should always be drawn off quickly once flow is established
    E Tapping at regular intervals is satisfactory

547. Regarding tuberculosis of the mesenteric lymph nodes in children:
    A Calcified lymph nodes on the mesentery seen on x-ray means the infection has been overcome
    B A differential diagnosis is non-specific mesenteric adenitis
    C The differential diagnosis from acute appendicitis may be almost impossible
    D Intestinal obstruction due to a caseating lymph node is an early complication
    E It is a cause of pseudomesenteric cyst

548. If a newborn infant is suffering from Hirschsprung's disease
- A the condition becomes apparent about three weeks after birth
- B the rectum feels empty and grips the examining finger
- C on withdrawing the examining finger from the anus there may be a short squirt of meconium
- D the caecum may perforate
- E total colectomy is necessary

549. The complications of typhoid infection include
- A paralytic ileus
- B intestinal haemorrhage
- C gallstone formation
- D osteomyelitis
- E laryngitis

550. If a woman aged 60 has diverticulitis of the sigmoid colon
- A she may have gallstones and an hiatus hernia
- B on a barium enema the condition is localised with no relaxation with Probanthine (propantheline)
- C bleeding is often periodic and profuse
- D she is likely to have a vesicovaginal fistula
- E excision of the affected area is the simplest method of treatment

551. Intestinal amoebiasis
- A is unknown in the United Kingdom
- B is due to the effects of *entamoeba coli*
- C can perforate the caecum
- D causes a carcinoma of the colon
- E causes a liver abscess which contains pus said to look like anchovy sauce

552. Crohn's disease
- A occurs mainly in old ladies
- B is common in the relatives of those who have ulcerative colitis
- C is restricted to the ileum, hence the term regional ileitis
- D should be called regional enteritis
- E involves mesenteric lymph nodes which contain Reed-Sternberg giant cells

553. In the operative assessment of a patient with carcinoma of the colon
- A the presence of secondary deposits in the liver is confirmed by palpation alone
- B the presence of secondary deposits in the liver is recorded following inspection as well as palpation
- C the presence of secondary deposits is a contraindication to resection of a carcinoma
- D the presence of enlarged lymph nodes confirms that spread has occurred
- E the liver is palpated before the growth

554. A patient with a faecal fistula in the right iliac fossa
- A which occurs after appendicectomy, may have actinomycosis
- B may be required to swallow a methylene blue tablet to prove the presence of the fistula
- C should be treated by an operation for closure of the fistula itself
- D should not be given anything by mouth
- E may require an ileostomy

555. Regarding gas shadows and fluid levels seen on an x-ray in cases of intestinal obstruction:
- A A fluid level seen at the duodenal cap is physiological
- B The distended jejunum is flat and characterless
- C The ileum is characterised by the concertina effect of the valvulae conniventes
- D Obstruction of the ascending colon often causes fluid levels in the small intestine despite the ileocaecal valve
- E The presence of fluid levels in the large intestine is an indication for an urgent barium meal and follow through

556. Regarding ileocolic intussusception:
- A The intussuscipiens is the apex of the intussusception
- B Gangrene is uncommon
- C It is the most uncommon form of intussusception
- D Clinically it can simulate gastroenteritis
- E Faecal matter and bile are present in all the stools

557. **Intestinal obstruction with strangulation of the blood vessels is caused by**
    A a band
    B a volvulus
    C an intussusception
    D Crohn's disease
    E acute enterocolitis

558. **Occlusion of the superior mesenteric artery**
    A may be due to fibrillation of the right atrium
    B may follow coronary thrombosis
    C may be due to thromboangiitis obliterans
    D is followed by an infarct
    E has only transient effects because there is a good collateral circulation

559. **The frequency with which the appendix lies in a particular position is**
    A subcaecal in 40%
    B retrocaecal in 30%
    C pelvic in 20%
    D pre-ileal in 1%
    E post-ileal in 15%

560. **Regarding appendicectomy for acute appendicitis:**
    A The incision should relate to the position in which the appendix is thought to lie
    B A Kocher's incision is useful for a pelvic appendix
    C It is not necessary to bury the stump of the appendix
    D Haemostasis is achieved by diathermy
    E The peritoneal cavity should be drained

561. **In a newborn child who has what is generally termed imperforate anus:**
    A It is due to agenesis or atresia of the rectum and anus
    B The child may have an ectopic anus
    C There may be a rectovesical fistula
    D Other congenital abnormalities may be present
    E A diagnostic perineal exploration suffices to solve the problem

562. Internal piles
- A contain veins, arteries and nerves
- B are often symptomatic of portal hypertension
- C are principally three in number located at 1, 5 and 7 o'clock with the patient in the lithotomy position
- D are the cause of proctalgia fugax
- E are called second degree when they are permanently prolapsed

563. The causes of proctitis include
- A piles
- B gonorrhoea
- C parasites
- D the *entamoeba histolytica*
- E a polypus

564. An ischiorectal abscess
- A is a perianal abscess
- B can be caused by a blood-borne infection
- C may be tuberculous in nature
- D can spread to the contralateral side
- E should be treated rigorously with antibiotics and local heat

565. Carcinoma of the rectum
- A is a nodule before it become an ulcer
- B may occur in a previously benign adenoma
- C spreads locally in a longitudinal manner
- D penetrates the fascia propria at an early stage
- E only exceptionally is there downward lymphatic spread

566. Infection of the umbilical cord
- A includes infection with streptococci
- B can cause an outbreak of puerperal sepsis
- C could be followed by neonatal tetanus
- D is a cause of jaundice in the newborn
- E is a cause of portal vein thrombosis

567. The contents of an inguinal hernial sac may include
- A an ovary
- B an appendix
- C a Meckel's diverticulum
- D a diverticulum of the bladder
- E omentum

568. In a patient with a strangulated Richter's hernia:
- A A portion of the circumference of the intestine is affected
- B It usually complicates a femoral hernia
- C The local signs of strangulation are often not obvious
- D Absolute constipation is pathognomonic
- E Vomiting is pathognomonic

569. Regarding operation for an indirect inguinal hernia:
- A It should not be performed on patients who have chronic bronchitis
- B General anaesthesia has to be used
- C In infants the posterior inguinal wall should be repaired
- D In adults the internal inguinal ring usually needs to be strengthened
- E Mesh implants may be used

570. A strangulated inguinal hernia
- A is tense
- B is tender
- C has a transmitted cough impulse
- D is irreducible
- E requires operation on the next operating list

571. In a 3-month old infant with an umbilical hernia:
- A The cause is usually sepsis of the cord
- B The hernia may become elongated and conical
- C Strangulation is likely to occur
- D Operation is necessary
- E The umbilicus should be excised

572. Regarding intravenous urography (I.V.P.):
- A It is contraindicated when the renal function is known to be poor
- B Sodium diatrizoate contains iodine
- C It is contraindicated in myelomatosis
- D Compression of the abdomen by a strap improves the emptying of the renal pelvis and therefore the x-ray visualisation
- E Residual urine cannot be demonstrated by this method

573. **Regarding congenital abnormalities of the kidney:**
   A In horseshoe kidney a urogram shows that the lowest calyx on each side is reversed
   B Patients with congenital cystic kidneys tend to pass small amounts of concentrated urine
   C Congenital cystic kidneys may present with uraemia
   D A solitary renal cyst is not always congenital
   E Aberrant renal vessels accentuate a hydronephrosis

574. **A patient with unilateral hydronephrosis**
   A has an incomplete urethral obstruction
   B may have an aberrant renal artery
   C may have a ureterocoele
   D is more likely to be a male
   E may suffer from Dietl's crisis

575. **If a patient is suffering from a stone passing down the ureter:**
   A The colic should be treated with sedatives
   B The topical application of a hot water bottle or heat pad suitably covered to protect the skin is of little value these days
   C The stone has to be removed later by the surgeon
   D Stone catchers and corkscrew stone dislodgers are useful for stones in the upper ureter
   E Ureteric meatotomy *via* an operating cystoscope is a commendable way of encouraging a stone to pass into the bladder

576. **If a patient has tuberculosis of the kidney:**
   A The patient is usually a woman of fifty years
   B The earliest symptom is haematuria
   C The urine is acid and contains pus cells
   D Changes in the pyelogram commence with loss or dysfunction of one or more calyces
   E Surgical procedures are now unnecessary because of advances in antituberculous chemotherapy

577. **Concerning tumours of the kidney:**
    A Benign tumours are rare
    B A nephroblastoma is a greyish white or pinkish white in colour
    C A hypernephroma is a big tumour which begins to grow at the upper pole of the kidney
    D Aortography shows an avascular area in the case of a tumour
    E Adequate treatment depends on nephrectomy and removal of the perinephric fat

578. **Regarding rupture of the bladder:**
    A It occurs intraperitoneally in 80% of cases
    B Intraperitoneal rupture is usually caused by a fractured pelvis
    C Most cases of extraperitoneal rupture cannot be differentiated from a rupture of the posterior urethra and the treatment is the same
    D Laparotomy is indicated for intraperitoneal rupture
    E If operation is delayed for more than twelve hours the mortality rises to over 50%

579. **Diverticulum of the bladder**
    A is usually congenital in origin
    B it is not lined by bladder mucosa
    C has no pathognomonic symptoms
    D may not be seen on cystoscopy
    E is removed when distal urinary obstruction is treated

580. **Regarding bilharziasis of the bladder:**
    A The *schistosoma haematobium* enters the body by being swallowed
    B The male worm is longer than the female
    C Urticaria is an early clinical feature
    D Women are more easily infected because of the shortness of the urethra
    E It can cause a squamous-celled carcinoma of the bladder

581. **In the diagnosis and management of malignant bladder tumours:**
    A A tumour nearly always presents with intermittent haematuria
    B An intravenous urogram is the mainstay of diagnosis
    C Assessment includes the use of the TNM classification
    D A small biopsy settles the diagnosis
    E The tumours are radio-insensitive

582. **Regarding the presentation of a benign enlargement of the prostate:**
   A Impotence is the rule in the early stages
   B The patient has to strain to pass urine
   C In acute retention of urine the urine is always infected
   D The prostate is incriminated if haematuria occurs
   E The urine may constantly dribble away

583. **Contracture of the bladder neck**
   A occurs in children of both sexes
   B affects women as well as men
   C can be due to muscle hypertrophy
   D presents as prostatism *sans* prostate
   E is treated by retropubic prostatectomy

584. **Concerning the natural history of carcinoma of the prostate:**
   A About 20% of cases of prostatic obstruction prove to be due to carcinoma
   B Tiny neoplasms found in serial sections of the prostate in 15% of men over fifty are examples of dormant cancer
   C The growth spreads early through the fascia of Denonvilliers
   D Bony metastases tend to be osteosclerotic
   E Lymph nodes do become involved

585. **Extravasation of urine in cases of complete rupture of the bulbous urethra**
   A cannot pass behind the mid-perineal point
   B can pass into the inguinal canals
   C can pass into the upper half of the thigh
   D cannot pass up the abdominal wall beneath the deep layer of the superficial fascia
   E can pass into the scrotum

586. **Gonorrhoea**
   A is due to the *Neisseria gonorrhoea* which is a gram positive coccus
   B can cause acute suppurative arthritis
   C can occur in the anus and rectum
   D begins by penetration by the gonococcus of the epithelium of the glans penis
   E often presents as acute retention of urine

587. Regarding balanoposthitis:
- A Inflammation of the prepuce is called posthitis
- B Inflammation of the glans is called balanitis
- C A cancer may be the cause of balanoposthitis
- D A chancre is not a cause of balanposthitis
- E Operation is unnecessary

588. Concerning lymphogranuloma inguinale:
- A The Frei test should be positive
- B It is due to Donovania granulomatis
- C The primary lesion is a vesicle surrounded by erythema looking a bright, beefy red
- D It is a cause of rectal stricture
- E It responds to sulphonamides

589. Regarding carcinoma of the penis:
- A Circumcision in childhood gives complete immunity against the condition
- B It is a disease of the elderly
- C Enlargement of the inguinal lymph nodes means that metastasis has taken place
- D Radiotherapy gives good results with small well-differentiated tumours
- E Total amputation of the penis means that the patient will have a perineal urethrostomy

590. Regarding torsion of the testis:
- A It is common
- B It is related to anomalies in the anchorage of the testis
- C If affecting an imperfectly descended testis it is difficult to distinguish it from a strangulated inguinal hernia
- D Excepting C (above) it cannot be confused with anything else
- E It requires treatment by bed rest and cold compresses

591. A varicocoele
- A usually occurs on the right side
- B feels, on standing, like a mass of worms
- C is best managed by wearing tight pants
- D causes oligospermia
- E may be operated upon if there is intractable cord pain

592. Cysts of the epididymis
A contain barley-water-like fluid
B are spermatocoeles
C are tense cysts
D are situated in front of the body of the testis
E may transilluminate like a Chinese lantern

593. Tuberculous epididymitis:
A Usually begins in the globus major
B Feels firm and craggy
C Is often associated with a thickened 'beaded' vas
D The testis is often involved by it
E The semen may yield tubercle bacilli on culture

594. Regarding neoplasm of the testis:
A A seminoma arises in the interstitial cells of the testis
B A teratoma arises from the mediastinum testis
C A Leydig-cell tumour arises from the rete testis
D The peak incidence of teratoma testis is between 20–25 years of age
E Macroscopically the seminoma is homogenous, pink or cream in colour

595. The action to be taken when the clinical diagnosis of neoplasm of the testis includes
A a chest x-ray
B orchiectomy (or exploration)
C dissection of inguinal lymph nodes
D vasectomy on the contralateral side
E radiotherapy

596. Concerning the management and prognosis of malignant tumours of the testis:
A 25% with seminoma without metastases survive five years if treated by orchiectomy and radiotherapy
B 80% with teratoma (differentiated) without metastases survive five years if treated by orchiectomy and radiotherapy
C Seminomas are highly radio-insensitive
D Radiotherapy should be given by a cobalt or linear accelerator x-ray unit
E An x-ray of the chest and an I.V.P. are essential in assessment before radiotherapy is given

597. Carcinoma of the scrotum
  A spreads to the inguinal lymph nodes (horizontal group)
  B develops from Cock's peculiar tumour
  C may occur in workers whose trousers tend to become soaked in lubricating oil
  D is a columnar celled carcinoma
  E is almost unknown in India and Asiatic countries

598. Successful kidney transplantation between a recipient and a living related donor depends upon
  A compatible ABO blood grouping
  B HLA (human leucocyte antigen) matching
  C a positive cytotoxic result of a cross match
  D an I.V.P. of the donor
  E an aortogram of the donor

599. In relation to kidney transplantation a prospective donor may be declared dead if
  A there is no spontaneous respiratory movement when the patient's CO_2 is normal
  B unequal pupils are present
  C one E.E.G. trace is flat on all channels
  D the diagnosis is made by the physician and not the surgeon involved in the case
  E if the patient is becoming hypothermic

600. In the management of a patient with a terminal illness
  A the correct dose of an analgesic for someone in pain is that dose which the patient says relieves the pain
  B the correct dose of an analgesic is the standard dose
  C the patient should be kept in bed
  D physiotherapy is no longer necessary and the patient should not be bothered with it
  E questions of escalating dosages of analgesics become irrelevant

PART III
SINGLE RESPONSE (1 IN 4) SET AT RANDOM

Questions requiring a single negative response are marked with an asterisk.

PART III

601. A greenstick fracture
 A occurs chiefly in the elderly
 B does not occur in children
 C is a spiral fracture of tubular bone
 D is a fracture where part of the cortex is intact and part is crumpled or cracked

602. Sympathetic ophthalmia is
 A conjunctivitis in both eyes due to injury
 B subconjunctival haemorrhage due to a fractured base of skull
 C infective (contagious) conjunctivitis
 D an autoimmune reaction causing blindness in a normal eye following injury of the other eye

603. A bunion is
 A an exostosis of the base of the first metatarsal
 B a type of sesamoid bone
 C an inflamed adventitious bursa beside the head of the first metatarsal
 D an exostosis of the head of the first metatarsal

604. A ruptured ear drum should be treated by
 A eardrops
 B daily examination
 C a grommet tube
 D myringotomy

605. The five-year survival rate after treatment of all varieties of carcinoma of the tongue is
 A 10%
 B 15%
 C 25%
 D 40%

606. Cock's peculiar tumour is synonymous with
 A rodent ulcer of the nose
 B local osteomyelitis of the cranium
 C chronic infection of a sebaceous cyst
 D keratin horn of the heel

607. Proud flesh is the term used to describe
   A excessive granulation tissue
   B muscle protruding through a skin wound
   C hypertrophy of the nose
   D hypertrophy of the tongue

608. A tuberculous ulcer has
   A a shelving edge
   B a rolled edge
   C an undermined edge
   D an everted edge

609. Lymph nodes draining a syphilitic chancre of the genitalia area are
   A bulky
   B soft
   C firm
   D cystic

610. A choledochus cyst is
   A congenital
   B parasitic
   C more common in males than in females
   D symptomless

*611. Pure cholesterol stones are
   A single
   B multiple
   C light in weight
   D radio-opaque

*612. In an attack of gallstone colic, the patient
   A lies still, afraid to move
   B is doubled up
   C may roll on the floor
   D if a woman, she would prefer having a baby

613. Courvoisier's Law concerns
   A the length of a skin flap in skin grafting
   B ureteric calculi
   C jaundice
   D portal hypertension

*614. **The Marseilles classification of pancreatitis includes**
   A relapsing acute pancreatitis
   B idiopathic pancreatitis
   C chronic pancreatitis
   D relapsing chronic pancreatitis

615. **Following an operation for hallux valgus, the most satisfied patients are those who had**
   A an associated hammer toe
   B pain
   C metatarsus primus varus
   D an associated bunionette

616. **Malunion of a fracture is**
   A a fracture which unites in a position of deformity
   B delayed union of a fracture
   C non-union of a fracture
   D followed by pseudoarthrosis

617. **Sudeck's atrophy is**
   A a form of pressure atrophy
   B due to ischaemia of muscles
   C a form of osteoporosis
   D due to a neuropathy

618. **Volkmann's contracture**
   A affects the palmar fascia
   B develops at the ankle in a case of chronic venous ulcer
   C follows ischaemia of the forearm muscles
   D is due to excessive scarring of the skin of the arm following a burn

619. **Antisepsis depends entirely upon**
   A carbolic acid
   B iodine
   C a commitment against all infection caused by trauma or operation
   D theatre ventilation

620. **In the healing of a wound the normal tensile strength of the tissues is regained in**
   A 2 weeks
   B 6 weeks
   C 6 months
   D 2 years

621. Ischaemia means
  A pain in the ischial tuberosities
  B anaemia due to malignant secondaries in the ischial part of the pelvis
  C lack of blood flow
  D increased blood flow

622. The venom of a wasp sting
  A is acid
  B remains in the avulsed venom gland of the wasp
  C is alkaline
  D is never dangerous

623. The special danger of a carotid body tumour is that
  A it recurs after excision
  B it is blended with the carotid artery
  C it is blended with the external jugular vein
  D it is radioresistant

*624. The disadvantage of using radio-iodine to treat thyrotoxicosis is that
  A drug therapy is prolonged
  B an indefinite follow up is essential
  C there is a progressive incidence of thyroid insufficiency
  D it should be avoided under the age of 45

625. Which of the following is not correct in the presentation of carcinoma of the thyroid?
  A Earache
  B Hoarseness of the voice
  C A pulsating bone tumour
  D The sex ratio is 3 males to 1 female

626. The term lateral aberrant thyroid implies
  A congenital aberrant thyroid tissue lateral to the thyroid
  B a metastasis in a cervical lymph node from an occult thyroid carcinoma
  C a metastasis from carcinoma of the larynx
  D a type of branchial cyst

627. Fat necrosis of the breast does not
   A occur because the patient also has acute pancreatitis
   B cause retraction of the nipple
   C follow a blow
   D occur in stout middle-aged women

628. The treatment of a breast abscess should depend upon
   A incision
   B excision
   C biopsy
   D antibiotics

629. Mondor's disease is
   A an obscure type of thrombophlebitis particularly affecting veins of the breast
   B lymphoedema of the arm
   C chondritis of a costal cartilage
   D pectus excavatum

*630. Non-malignant conditions of the breast include
   A cystosarcoma phylloides
   B duct ectasia
   C giant fibroadenoma
   D Paget's disease of the nipple

631. An influence for good in managing a patient with intermittent claudication is
   A exercise
   B smoking
   C sugar
   D steroids

632. A mycotic aneurysm from the teleological point of view should be related only to
   A bacterial infection
   B fungal infection
   C the retinal vessels
   D the tympanic artery

633. The Hunterian ligature operation is performed for
   A varicose veins
   B arteriovenous fistula
   C an aneurysm
   D a lymph fistula

634. In the Matas operation what is reconstructed?
A An artery
B A vein
C A nerve
D A joint

635. A mallet finger is
A a swollen finger caused by a blow with a hammer or mallet
B an avulsion fracture of the extensor tendon to the proximal phalanx
C an avulsion fracture of the distal phalanx at the attachment of the long flexor tendon
D an avulsion fracture of the terminal slip of the extensor tendon to the distal phalanx

636. The safest form of treatment of fracture of the tibia and fibula is
A by plaster with manipulative reduction
B by skeletal traction
C by internal fixation with plates and screws
D by intramedullary nailing

637. Regarding a torn meniscus of the knee:
A It is usually the lateral meniscus
B It is not uncommon in women
C It occurs when the foot is fixed and the knee is slightly bent and the body falls forward
D It occurs when the foot is fixed, the knee is slightly bent and the body is twisted

638. Operative control of bleeding from wounds or incision of the scalp is best achieved by
A direct pressure applied to the skin
B diathermy to bleeding vessels
C eversion of the galea aponeurotica
D applying several forceps to the bleeding points

639. The serum of a patient with red cell group AB contains
A anti A and B antibody
B anti B antibody
C anti A antibody
D no AB antibody

640. If hepatitis follows blood transfusion it occurs
  A one week later
  B one month later
  C three months later
  D six months later

641. Allowing blood which is ready for transfusion to remain for four hours in a warm environment
  A reduces shock
  B increases shock
  C favours subsequent hepatitis
  D encourages bacterial proliferation and septicaemia

642. Christmas disease is
  A haemophilia B (Factor IX deficiency)
  B haemolysis of blood cells due to severe cold
  C haemophilia A (Factor VIII deficiency)
  D hypercoagulability due to cold

643. The initial abnormality in rheumatoid arthritis is
  A fibrillation of cartilage
  B sclerosis of cartilage
  C in the synovial membrane
  D in the capsule

644. In ankylosing spondylitis the most affected joint in the following list is the
  A sacro-iliac joint
  B shoulder joint
  C sterno-clavicular joint
  D hip joint

645. In the operation of arthroplasty
  A only the joint is excised and the two ends are brought into apposition to obtain fusion
  B only the capsule of the joint is reefed in order to strengthen the joint
  C only the joint is excised without bringing the bone ends together to obtain fusion
  D only the diseased synovial membrane is removed

646. An ecchondroma
   A grows in the medulla of bone
   B grows on the surface of bone
   C is due to rickets
   D often undergoes malignant change if the tumour is solitary

647. The weight of patients subsisting entirely on parenteral fluids should
   A gain 100–200 g per day
   B keep weight steady
   C lose 100–200 g per day
   D lose 300–500 g per day

648. Respiratory arrest due to respiratory alkalosis is rectified by
   A insufflation with carbon dioxide
   B insufflation with oxygen
   C insufflation with helium
   D immediate tracheotomy

649. The acute acidosis which occurs after releasing a cross-clamped aorta (during operation for aneurysm), or in cardiac arrest requires the infusion of
   A 25 ml 6·4% sodium bicarbonate
   B 50–150 mEq 6·4% sodium bicarbonate
   C 50–150 mmol 8·4% sodium bicarbonate
   D 150–250 ml 10% sodium bicarbonate

650. The normal arterial PCO$_2$ is
   A 4·1–5·6 kPa
   B 15–25 mmHg
   C 7·1–10·5 kPa
   D 40–50 mmHg

651. Aniline, bilharzia, magenta and exfoliative cytology are related in terms of
   A carcinoma of the colon
   B carcinoma of the cervix
   C bronchial tumours
   D bladder tumours

*652. **The boundaries of the inguinal canal include**
   A   anteriorly-transversalis fascia
   B   posteriorly-conjoined tendon
   C   superiorly-conjoined muscles
   D   inferiorly-inguinal ligament

653. **Cholangitis is**
   A   thrombophlebitis of small hepatic veins
   B   pyelophlebitis
   C   inflammation of the bile ducts
   D   the 'cardiac link' between the heart and the gallbladder

654. **Dysphagia lusoria is due to**
   A   an oesophageal diverticulum
   B   oesophageal webs
   C   an aneurysm of the aorta
   D   an abnormal arrangement of the arch of the aorta

655. **Which of the following is incorrect?**
   A   Secondary deposits in the spine far outnumber spinal cord tumours
   B   Extradural tumours are usually meningiomas or neurofibromas
   C   Intramedullary tumours are usually gliomas or ependymomas
   D   The majority of secondary deposits in the spine are derived from bronchial carcinoma

656. **Regarding causalgia which of the following is incorrect?**
   A   It tends to follow complete nerve injury
   B   A lateral neuroma may be present
   C   A histamine-like substance produces the physical signs
   D   Paravertebral block may give relief

657. **Which of the following is the most important in the management of boils and 'pimples' in the mask area of the face?**
   A   Dressings with magnesium sulphate and glycerine paste
   B   Short wave diathermy
   C   A broad spectrum antibiotic
   D   Avoidance of squeezing or pricking the lesion

658. **Regarding acute empyema of the antrum one of the following is incorrect?**
   A   Pain is sometimes referred along one of the trigeminal nerve
   B   Treatment includes ephedrine 1% in saline by a nebulizer
   C   X-ray reveals a relative translucency of the affected antrum
   D   Puncturing of the antrum is for diagnostic and therapeutic purposes

659. **Which of the following clinical features is not related to hyperparathyroidism?**
   A   Risus sardonicus
   B   Psychic moans
   C   Abdominal groans
   D   Pain from renal stones

660. **Regarding Addison's disease, which of the following is incorrect?**
   A   It is due to acute cortical haemorrhage of the adrenals
   B   Tuberculosis accounts for 50% of cases
   C   The medulla may not be implicated
   D   A leading feature is muscular weakness

661. **Regarding Conn's syndrome, which of the following is incorrect?**
   A   It is due to a common adrenocortical tumour producing aldosterone
   B   There is sodium retention
   C   There is oliguria
   D   There is polydipsia

662. **Which is incorrect about ganglioneuroma? It**
   A   is relatively benign
   B   grows to a large size
   C   never involves the adrenal gland
   D   constitutes one of the variety of retroperitoneal tumours

663. **The foramen of Bochdalek occurs in**
   A   the base of the skull
   B   the heart
   C   the diaphragm
   D   the pelvis

*664. In a patient with retrosternal goitre:
   A   It is frequently bilateral
   B   Calcification is common
   C   Scabbard trachea can occur
   D   The blood supply is thoracic and a sternal splitting approach is necessary

665. Which of the following is not a mediastinal cyst?
   A   Spring water cyst
   B   'Water lily' cyst
   C   Foregut cyst
   D   Pleuropericardial

*666. The immediate treatment of cardiac arrest includes
   A   closed cardiac massage
   B   keeping the patient fully supine
   C   the correction of metabolic acidosis
   D   maintaining a good airway

667. Which one of these statements is true in the diagnosis of congenital dislocation of the hip in the first few days of life?
   A   It is impossible to diagnose it
   B   The sign of telescoping is the best way of diagnosing it
   C   It is possible to diagnose it by the Van Rosen/Barlow Test
   D   The Trendelenberg test is the most useful

668. If an unstable hip is detected at birth the management policy is
   A   do nothing and re-examine every six months as only a minority of hips develop into a persistent dislocation
   B   use a splint to keep the hip joint in 45° flexion and adduction
   C   use a splint to keep the hip joint in 90° flexion and abduction
   D   advise operative stabilisation

669. Shenton's line is a sign applicable to
   A   the detection of shortening of the leg on physical examination
   B   a radiological feature of the pelvis applied to the diagnosis of congenital dislocation of the hip
   C   a radiological feature of the lungs applied to the diagnosis of pulmonary vein thrombosis
   D   a physical sign applied to the diagnosis of adrenal deficiency

670. **Which is inappropriate to surgical treatment of the hip in a child of six with congenital dislocation of the hip?**
    A Pelvic osteotomy
    B Shelf operation
    C McMurray's osteotomy
    D Intertrochanteric rotation osteotomy of the femur

671. **Excessive distension of the small intestine in intestinal obstruction may require relief by**
    A gastrostomy by trochar and cannula through the abdominal wall
    B a Celestin tube
    C a Savage type intestinal decompressor at laparotomy
    D a Fogarty catheter at laparotomy

*672. **Volvulus of the intestine**
    A can affect the new born
    B can be caecal
    C may require a Paul-Mikulicz procedure
    D is unknown in India

673. **Which is the only acceptable solution here for the injection of haemorrhoids?**
    A 5% sodium tetradecyl sulphate
    B 5% phenol in almond or arachis oil
    C 5% phenol in water
    D Pure almond or arachis oil

674. **The following, save one, simulate external haemorrhoids:**
    A Anal warts
    B Condylomas
    C Hypertrophic tuberculide
    D Leucoplakia

675. **An adventitious bursa is**
    A an anatomical bursa overlying any joint
    B a type of degeneration of the adventitia of the popliteal artery
    C an acquired bursa generated from connective tissue
    D a pseudocyst in the lesser sac (omental bursa)

676. **In the management of paralysis which of the following principles is undesirable?**
   A The re-establishment of joint stability by operation or splinting
   B Allowing flexor and adductor muscle groups to overcome extensors
   C Reinforcing paralysed groups
   D Weakening non-paralysed groups

677. **Which of the following nouns is associated with joint neuropathy?**
   A Hutchinson
   B Hutchison
   C Moon
   D Charcot

678. **Bennetts fracture is**
   A a reversed Colles' fracture
   B a fracture of the scaphoid bone in the wrist
   C a fracture of the radial styloid (chauffeur's fracture)
   D a fracture dislocation of the first metacarpal

679. **Of a march fracture which statement is incorrect?**
   A It is the result of anaemia and general fatigue
   B It may not show up on immediate x-ray
   C It is the result of localised stress and fatigue
   D In the foot it is predisposed to by a short first metatarsal

*680. **Villous adenomas of the rectum**
   A can be treated by local excision
   B may be very large
   C can cause hypokalaemia
   D are always benign

681. **The site of the neck of a femoral hernia is**
   A the transversalis fascia
   B the iliopectineal ligament
   C the femoral ring
   D the cribriform fascia

*682. **Stones which form in an acid urine include those composed of**
   A   oxalate
   B   cystin
   C   calcium ammonia magnesium phosphate
   D   urate

*683. **A vesical calculus may be composed of**
   A   oxalate
   B   uric acid
   C   triple phosphate
   D   calcium bilirubinate

684. **Aneurysmal bone cysts:**
   A   Are true aneurysms of nutrient arteries
   B   Occur only in flat bones
   C   Are the same as osseous haemangiomas
   D   Are almost certainly not neoplastic

685. **A giant cell tumour of bone shows on x-ray**
   A   sun ray spicules
   B   Codman's triangle
   C   a soap bubble appearance
   D   shotty calcification

686. **Radiotherapy for osteosarcoma means a dose in the region of**
   A   1000 rad only
   B   3000 rad in divided doses over one month
   C   6000 rad over one month
   D   9000 rad over three months

687. **The reported incidence of unstable hips at birth is as much as**
   A   1 per 10000
   B   2–4 per 1000
   C   8–20 per 1000
   D   28–40 per 1000

688. **In retrosternal goitre which of the following is correct?**
   A   A ^{127}I scan may help to distinguish a retrosternal from a mediastinal tumour
   B   Dysphagia is common
   C   Recurrent nerve paralysis is common
   D   It may be malignant

689. Wayne's clinical diagnostic index is used in the diagnosis of
 A phaeochromocytoma
 B an insulinoma
 C thyrotoxicosis
 D Zollinger-Ellison syndrome

690. Wharton's duct drains
 A the pancreas
 B the parotid
 C the lacrymal gland
 D the submandibular gland

691. Which of the following is not included in the triad of Mikulicz?
 A Symmetrical enlargement of all the salivary glands
 B Narrowing of the palpebral fissures
 C Dryness of the mouth
 D Rheumatoid arthritis

692. Regarding cervical rib, which statement is correct?
 A It always connects to the scalene tubercle by a fibrous band
 B It passes through the apex of the supraclavicular triangle
 C It causes pressure on the ulnar nerve
 D Pain is often located in the forearm

693. In Boeck's sarcoidosis which of the following is common?
 A Fever
 B Erythema nodosum
 C Pulmonary infiltration followed by hilar adenopathy
 D Secondary infections

694. A pulp abscess of a finger should be drained by
 A a long incision in the long axis of the pulp
 B an incision right across the volar aspect of the pulp
 C a small incision at the point of maximum tenderness without deeper exploration
 D a small incision designed to uncap the abscess at the point of maximum tenderness with examination for and removal of any deeper slough

695. **Kanavel's sign is**
    A swelling above the flexor retinaculum
    B flexion of the thumb when the radial bursa is infected
    C flexion of the fingers in a compound palmar ganglion
    D tenderness over an infected ulnar bursa between the transverse palmar creases

696. **The space of Parona is**
    A in the wrist between the deep flexor tendons and the pronator quadratus
    B above the patella between the quadriceps muscle and the femur
    C beneath the tendon of the iliopsoas
    D between the Achilles tendon and the posterior aspect of the tibia

697. **Grey-Turner sign in acute pancreatitis is**
    A discoloration in the loins
    B shifting dullness over the spleen
    C discoloration around the umbilicus
    D a fluid level in the first loop of the jejunum

698. **Secondary malignant deposits observed in the peritoneal cavity can, with one exception, be confused with**
    A peritoneal hydatids
    B tuberculous peritonitis
    C fat necrosis
    D pneumococcal peritonitis

*699. **Regarding ulcerative colitis:**
    A The cause is unknown
    B The disease starts in the rectum and spreads proximally in 95% of cases
    C Pan-procto colectomy is appropriate
    D Acne is a related lesion

700. **Cramer wire is used**
    A for wiring the patella
    B for repairing a hernia by darning
    C as a splint
    D to transfix bone for traction purposes

701. When anaesthetising for an infected index finger one of the following is contraindicated:
    A A rubber tourniquet
    B 2% xylocaine
    C 0·5% adrenaline
    D A 'ring' block

702. Orf is
    A a fungus infection of the nail bed
    B a virus disease of sheep which can occur on the fingers
    C an infected ganglion
    D a pilonidal sinus between the fingers of barbers

703. Madura foot is
    A an infection caused by a type of monilia
    B a swelling due to a stress fracture of the second metatarsal
    C an infection caused by a type of actinomyces
    D a swelling due to an infected perforating ulcer

704. The normal arterial PO_2 is
    A 30–40 mmHg
    B 6·1–7·16 kPa
    C 80–110 mmHg
    D 15·5–20 kPa

705. A patient with a pH 7·30, PCO_2 60 mmHg, Base excess +1 has
    A uncompensated respiratory acidosis
    B severe metabolic acidosis
    C compensatory metabolic alkalosis
    D metabolic alkalosis

706. 'Carbohydrate provides the fire in which fat is burnt', so when fat is used as a source of calories it is necessary that
    A 15% of the total should be carbohydrate
    B 20% of the total should be carbohydrate
    C 30% of the total should be carbohydrate
    D 40% of the total should be carbohydrate

707. The desirable calorie intake by parenteral nutrition alone is
    A 500–1000
    B 1000–1500
    C 1500–2000
    D at least 2000

708. **A keratin horn**
    A arises from a sebaceous cyst
    B is due to matting of hair
    C is a papilloma with excess keratin formation
    D is congenital

709. **Concerning the pathology of craniocerebral injury which of these statements is incorrect?**
    A The brain is a perfect fit within its membranes
    B In deaths from boxing injuries the medulla may be torn across
    C Loss of consciousness is produced by paralysis of conduction in the brain stem
    D In cerebral contusion the stretch effect is severe

710. **A Pott's puffy tumour is**
    A an indurated chronically infected sebaceous cyst of the scalp
    B a swollen ankle due to a fracture of the lateral malleolus
    C localised pitting oedema of the scalp over an area of oestomyelitis of the scalp
    D a pulsating secondary deposit of the scalp from an hypernephroma

711. **Regarding chromophobe adenomas, which statement is incorrect? They**
    A are most common in men
    B are slow growing
    C may undergo involution
    D stretch the optic nerves to produce primary optic atrophy

712. **The cold water treatment of burns is applicable**
    A to the treatment of deep burns to encourage sloughs to separate
    B to the treatment of superficial burns as an alternative to the exposure method
    C as a first aid measure
    D for washing all burns on arrival at hospital

713. **A Thiersch graft is**
    A a partial thickness skin graft
    B a pinch skin graft
    C a small full thickness skin graft
    D a pedicle graft

714. **Tulle gras is**
    A a type of silk used in dressings
    B puckering of the skin around a carcinoma
    C a mesh type of dressing impregnated with some kind of petroleum jelly
    D a type of linen suture

715. **Chemical sympathectomy is effected by using**
    A 5% phenol solution in arachis oil
    B 10% phenol solution in olive oil
    C 12% phenol in water
    D 5% phenol solution in water

*716. **Sliding hiatus hernia**
    A is acquired
    B is part of Saint's triad
    C accounts for 20% of cases of hiatus hernia
    D is the cause of 'congenital short oesophagus'.

*717. **In carcinoma of the oesophagus**
    A 50% of the lesions involve the middle third
    B about 30% of the patients are women
    C from the beginning there is dysphagia to liquids as well as solids
    D spread by the blood stream is exceptional

*718. **Regarding gastrin:**
    A It is released in response to mechanical distension of the antrum
    B It is released by the G-cell and reaches the parietal cell by the local splanchnic circulation
    C There is more than one gastrin
    D Its release stimulates gastric motor activity by a slight increase in slow wave frequency and a marked increase in associated contractile activity

*719. **Acute peptic ulcers**
    A seldom invade the muscle layer
    B can occur anywhere in the stomach
    C present with haemorrhage
    D are rarely multiple

720. A Milwaukee brace is used in
- A sacro-iliac strain
- B derangement of the teeth
- C a patient with an above knee amputation
- D scoliosis

721. A slipped femoral epiphysis
- A is due to infarction of the epiphysis
- B occurs in overweight multipara
- C occurs in overweight boys between 10–18 years
- D affects overweight girls between 4–8 years

722. Tennis elbow is
- A olecranon bursitis
- B 'non-articular rheumatism' of the attachment of the extensor muscles of the forearm to the lateral epicondyle of the humerus
- C 'non-articular rheumatism' of the attachment of the flexor muscles to the medial epicondyle
- D myositis ossificans of the supinator

723. A trigger finger is
- A a sore index finger
- B an atrophic index finger of a median nerve palsy
- C due to stenosing tenovaginitis affecting one of the flexor tendons in the palm
- D an essential part of the carpal tunnel syndrome

*724. Coarctation of the aorta
- A may occur at any site
- B usually occurs above the origin of the left subclavian artery
- C is a cause of intermittent claudication
- D causes headaches

725. Regarding ventricular septal defect, which statement is incorrect? It
- A may be part of Fallot's tetralogy
- B causes overfilling of the right heart
- C is the rarest of congenital cardiac anomalies
- D results in 50% mortality in the first few months of life

*726. Mitral valvotomy for mitral stenosis
  A is best performed between the ages of 20–50 years
  B should be considered when the symptoms are aggravated by pregnancy
  C is not indicated in persistent congestive heart failure
  D gives good results when the mitral valve is immobile

727. Regarding oesophagitis, which is inappropriate?
  A Scalds
  B Acid reflux
  C Alkaline reflux
  D Anaemia is uncommon

728. Denis Browne splints are used in the management of
  A undescended testicle
  B cleft palate
  C talipes
  D fractured os calcis

729. Congenital torticollis is due to
  A a rhabdomyoma of the sternomastoid
  B infarction of the sternomastoid at birth
  C a hemi-cervical vertebra
  D failure of the clavicle to develop

730. The essential examination of the hip in order to clinch the diagnosis of chronic slipped femoral epiphysis is
  A measuring for shortening of the leg
  B palpation of the femoral head
  C A-P plain x-ray view of the hip
  D lateral x-ray view of the hip

731. Osgood-Schlatter's disease is
  A a traction injury of the femoral epiphysis
  B A traction injury of the tibial tubercle of the tibial epiphysis
  C a traction injury of the posterior epiphysis of the os calcis
  D a traction injury of vertebral epiphysis

732. Regarding operation for duodenal ulceration:
  A Early operation gives the best results
  B It is indicated for hourglass deformity
  C The risks of operation far outweigh the risks of having an ulcer for five years
  D The patient should 'earn' his operation

*733. **Regarding hourglass stomach:**
   A   It mostly occurs in men
   B   It is usually silent
   C   A Billroth I gastrectomy is required
   D   Weight loss is very great

734. **Which of the following is not related clinically or pathologically to carcinoma of the stomach?**
   A   Blood group O
   B   Troisier's sign
   C   Linitis plastica
   D   Krukenberg tumours

735. **The prognosis following resection of carcinoma of the stomach is determined by**
   A   the extent of stomach removed
   B   the margin of apparently healthy stomach removed above the growth
   C   a short clinical history
   D   the histology of the growth

736. **Which of the following macroscopic characteristics of a cancer of the breast is incorrect?**
   A   The growth may grate whilst being cut
   B   Both surfaces are usually concave
   C   The colour of the cut surface is grey
   D   It will be found that there are remains of a capsule

737. **Of the operations listed, the interests of a patient with a Stage III carcinoma of the breast are best served by**
   A   a radical mastectomy
   B   a super-radical mastectomy
   C   simple mastectomy
   D   lumpectomy

738. **Gynaecomazia is not**
   A   an abnormal enlargement of the female breast
   B   associated with leprosy
   C   encountered in patients with Klinefelter's syndrome
   D   associated with liver failure

739. The indications for tonsillectomy do not include
- A enlarged tonsils
- B one attack of peritonsillar abscess
- C chronic tonsillitis
- D biopsy for suspected malignancy

740. Immediately after operation body potassium is
- A retained in the body
- B is increasingly excreted
- C is exchanged for calcium
- D is exchanged for magnesium

741. Darrow's solution does not contain
- A sodium
- B chloride
- C bicarbonate
- D lactate

742. Ringer lactate solution does not contain
- A sodium
- B chloride
- C bicarbonate
- D potassium

743. Using a plastic transfusion set the maintenance dose rate for intravenous fluid is about
- A 15 drips/min
- B 30 drips/min
- C 60 drips/min
- D 90 drips/min

744. The following, except one, are correct regarding malignant tumours of the nasopharynx:
- A Most of the growth arises in the supratonsillar fossa of Rosenmüller
- B In the U.K. it occurs especially where furniture is made
- C It does not involve cranial nerves
- D By the time a diagnosis is made 70% of the patients have enlarged cervical nodes

745. Concerning the value of tracheostomy, which statement is incorrect?
- A It allows assisted respiration in respiratory paralysis
- B It increases the anatomical dead space
- C It relieves obstruction of the upper air passages
- D It enables effective aspiration of the bronchus to be done

*746. Regarding bilateral recurrent laryngeal palsy:
  A It is a complication of thyroidectomy
  B The cords tend to get sucked together on expiration
  C Tracheostomy is necessary
  D Asphyxia and death may follow

*747. Regarding carcinoma of the larynx:
  A It is more common than an innocent tumour of the larynx
  B 70% arise from the true vocal cord
  C That arising in the false vocal cords has the worst prognosis
  D Women are ten times more often affected than men

*748. Regarding testicular tumour:
  A It can simulate epidydymo-orchitis
  B The lymphatic drainage is to the inguinal lymph nodes
  C It is painful in about 30% of cases
  D The left supraclavicular fossa is included in the examination

749. Ludwig's angina is due to
  A a type of coronary artery spasm
  B oesophageal spasm
  C retropharyngeal infection
  D a virulent infection of the cellular tissues around the submandibular salivary gland

750. The Cimino shunt is an arteriovenous fistula
  A external at the ankle
  B external at the wrist
  C internal at the thigh
  D internal at the wrist

751. 'Idiopathic' adult flat foot is primarily due to
  A collapse of lateral longitudinal arch
  B overstretched plantar ligaments
  C collapse of the medial longitudinal arch
  D a congenital bar of bone between the talus and the navicular bones

752. The nerve of Kuntz is an important landmark in
  A lumbar sympathectomy
  B cervicodorsal sympathectomy
  C obturator neurectomy
  D splanchnicectomy

753. **In the management of phantom pain one of the following is not advisable:**
    A Reassurance that the feeling of a painful phantom limb will disappear in time
    B Proceeding with post-amputation exercises
    C Proceeding with limb fitting
    D Discussing phantom pain with students and nurses in front of the patient

754. **Ainhum is a lesion which is**
    A a type of anal fissure
    B a fibromatous polyp at the anal margin
    C mycotic infection of the heel
    D a fibrotic process affecting a toe

755. **A white leg is due to**
    A femoral deep vein thrombosis
    B lymphatic obstruction
    C femoral vein thrombosis and lymphatic obstruction
    D vena cava thrombosis and lymphatic obstruction

756. **If a patient is seen within 48 hours of the appearance of symptoms of osteomyelitis**
    A antibiotic treatment should be started immediately
    B antibiotic treatment should not be started until pus has formed, drainage carried out and culture and sensitivity obtained
    C antibiotic treatment should await the result of blood culture
    D chloramphenicol is the most suitable antibiotic

757. **Which of the following organisms might not be found in a patient with acute suppurative arthritis of the knee?**
    A *Mycobacterium tuberculosis*
    B *Neisseria gonococi*
    C Typhoid
    D Pneumococci

758. **Pott's paraplegia is due to**
    A haematomyelia following trauma
    B damage to the cord by bone when vertebrae collapse in tuberculosis of the spine
    C tuberculous pus and angulation in tuberculosis of the spine
    D damage to the corda equina after a fall

759. **A patient with bony ankylosis of the knee has**
    A   pain
    B   spasm of the muscles around the knee
    C   muscle wasting around the knee
    D   a slight degree of movement in the joint

760. **Which sclerosant is quite unacceptable as an injection for varicose veins?**
    A   Sodium tetradecyl sulphate
    B   Ethanolamine oleate
    C   Phenol 5% in arachis oil
    D   Lithium salicylate 30%

761. **Bisgaard treatment refers to that of**
    A   ruptured tendo Achilles
    B   venous ulcer
    C   an ischaemic (arterial) ulcer
    D   an ingrowing toenail

762. **For lymphography of the leg the lymphatics of the foot are first outlined by**
    A   direct injection of ultrafluid lipiodol (radio-opaque solution)
    B   direct injection of Hypaque (sodium diatrizoate)
    C   direct injection of patent blue dye on the dorsum of the foot
    D   subdermal injection of patent blue dye between the toes

763. **Which of the following is inappropriate in the investigation of Hodgkin's disease?**
    A   Intravenous urography
    B   Laparotomy
    C   Mediastinal scanning
    D   Kveim-Siltzbach test

764. **Radiotherapy for reticulosis means**
    A   a single dose of 500–1000 rad
    B   a single dose of 1500–2000 rad
    C   2500–3000 rad in divided doses
    D   3500–4000 rad in divided doses

*765. **Tracheal stenosis**
    A   is usually caused by intra-tracheal tumours
    B   commonly follows tracheostomy at the site of the inflatable cuff
    C   can be treated by resection of the trachea
    D   is a complication of tuberculosis

766. **Pancoast syndrome includes (with one exception)**
    A rib erosion
    B upper brachial plexus lesion
    C Horner's syndrome
    D an apical lung shadow

767. **The following, save one, are considered to be contraindications to radical resection of lung cancer**
    A Evidence of involvement of the oesophagus
    B Distant metastases
    C Generalised arterial disease
    D All patients over 65 years

768. **The cause of pyrexia within 48 hours of an operation is most likely to be any of the following save one:**
    A Urinary infection
    B Atelectasis
    C The trauma of the operation
    D Sepsis

*769. **The effects of splenectomy include**
    A changes in the bone marrow
    B hypertrophy of any splenunculi
    C eosinophilia
    D leucopaenia

*770. **Cysts of the spleen can be**
    A dermoid
    B choledochal
    C hydatid
    D traumatic

771. **Haemobilia is**
    A bilharzia in the blood
    B blood and bile in the peritoneal cavity
    C blood in the bile duct
    D bile fistula into the hepatic venous system

*772. **Oesophageal varices**
    A are restricted to the oesophagus
    B can be demonstrated by splenic-portography
    C can always be demonstrated by oesophagoscopy
    D can be treated by injection

*773. Portasystemic shunting operations are contraindicated
A if the patient's serum albumin is more than 40 g/litre
B if there is massive ascites
C if oesophageal varices have not bled
D if the patient has significant jaundice

774. A 'stove in' chest is not
A caused by a compression injury
B associated with paradoxical movement
C ever reduced by positive pressure ventilation
D treated by surgical correction if severe

*775. Shock lung
A is an uncommon complication after major trauma
B causes depression of gas exchange
C decreases the lung compliance
D means micro-thrombo-embolism of small lung vessels

776. In Tietze's disease
A there is a small retromammary fibroadenoma
B there is a painful swelling of the second costal cartilage
C the swelling should be explored
D x-ray shows circumscribed calcification

777. Which statement is incorrect about an haemothorax?
A The treatment aim is to remove the blood completely by aspiration
B Massive clotting frequently occurs
C Blood is a pleural irritant and causes pain and effusion
D No cause may be found

778. One of the following is not a sign of increasing blood loss:
A Increasing pallor
B Restlessness
C Shallow slow breathing
D Increasing pulse rate

779. The first aid treatment of ruptured varicose veins at the ankle includes
A keeping the patient in the sitting position
B applying a tourniquet
C direct pressure on the bleeding point
D applying two tourniquets

780. **A stab wound of the common femoral vein is**
    A easy to control
    B unimportant
    C serious
    D controlled by a tourniquet

781. **Blood for transfusion should be stored at**
    A −20°C
    B −4°C to 0°C
    C +2°C to +7°C
    D +10°C to +14°C

782. **A Fogarty catheter is designed to be used for**
    A draining the bladder
    B ureteric catheterisation
    C removing blood clot from arteries
    D arteriography

783. **A contraindication to elective arterial by-pass operations is evidence of**
    A diabetes
    B mild heart failure
    C Paget's disease
    D coronary thrombosis six months previously

784. **Of a knitted Dacron artery graft which statement is correct?**
    A It is not porous
    B It is eventually dissolved by tissue reaction
    C It never gets infected
    D It can be easily incised and the opening resutured

785. **Temporal arteritis is**
    A a local collagen disease
    B Takayasu's arteriopathy
    C a variety of Buerger's disease
    D temporary arterial spasm

786. **Broder's grading of malignant tumours depends on**
    A the degree of spread of tumour in the lymphatics
    B the degree of differentiation shown by component cells as viewed through the microscope
    C a clinical grading for carcinoma of the breast
    D an operative grading for carcinoma of the colon

787. **An hamartoma is**
   A any collection of blood clot
   B a haemorrhagic cyst of the thigh
   C a developmental malformation
   D a tumour of muscle

788. **A sequestration dermoid cyst is**
   A due to squamous cells being driven in by a needle
   B due to cells being buried during development
   C an example of parthenogenesis
   D a variety of sebaceous cyst

789. **Which of the following should not be included in the treatment of bacteraemic shock?**
   A Early hydrocortisone
   B Blood volume replacement
   C Prolonged administration of noradrenaline
   D Full doses of a broad spectrum antibiotic

790. **Insensible loss of fluid from skin and lungs for 24 hours is normally in the span of**
   A 100–250 ml
   B 250–500 ml
   C 500–750 ml
   D 750–1000 ml

791. **In SI units milli-equivalents/litre are replaced by**
   A millimoles per 100 ml
   B milligrams per 100 ml
   C millimoles per 1000 ml
   D milligrams per 1000 ml

792. **The powerful conservator of sodium is**
   A testosterone
   B progesterone
   C aldosterone
   D hydrocortisone

793. **The potassium a normal adult ingests each day is**
   A 2–3 g
   B 5–6 g
   C 8–10 g
   D over 10 g

794. **Granuloma pyogenicum should be treated by**
    A cauterisation
    B antibiotic ointment
    C excision
    D radiotherapy

795. **Bowen's disease of the skin is**
    A a complication of a sebaceous cyst
    B a tumour of sweat glands
    C a premalignant intradermal condition
    D a type of dermatitis

796. **The treatment of a primary malignant melanoma of the skin is**
    A wide excision
    B radiotherapy
    C cytotoxic therapy
    D immunotherapy

797. **A partial thickness burn of the skin**
    A is sensitive
    B is insensitive
    C requires a split skin graft
    D will separate as a slough in 2–3 weeks

798. **Which of the following in the management of extensive burns shock is not useful?**
    A Nasogastric tube
    B Blood transfusion
    C Morphine
    D Dextran 40

799. **A hypertrophic scar**
    A is the same as a keloid scar
    B requires radiotherapy for a cure
    C is simply a raised red scar which persists for a year or two before becoming white
    D only occurs on the abdomen

800. **The best site for an intramuscular injection is**
    A the abdomen
    B the forearm
    C the inner lower quadrant of the buttock
    D the outer upper quadrant of the buttock

PART IV
DETERMINATE RESPONSE (YES AND NO) SET AT RANDOM

PART II

PART IV

801. Methods of wound closure to achieve protection by skin cover include
  A secondary suture
  B skin grafting
  C plaster of Paris cast
  D delayed primary suture
  E plastic spray

802. The staphylococcus aureus
  A is gram negative
  B forms chains
  C can live in the nostrils
  D is the usual cause of tonsillitis
  E forms penicillinase

803. Amyloid disease
  A is not a malignant disease
  B may be diagnosed on rectal biopsy
  C can occur in chronic osteomyelitis
  D is stained by osmic acid
  E is treated with ethambutol

804. The symptoms of occlusive vascular disease of the lower aorta may include
  A intermittent claudication
  B pain down the back of the leg at rest
  C pain in the foot at rest
  D pain in the knee joint
  E 'pins and needles' in the feet

805. An obstructed hernia
  A is irreducible
  B is strangulated
  C may be called 'incarcerated' when colon within the sac is blocked with faeces
  D can be caused by a truss
  E requires priority on the waiting list for elective surgery

806. The differential diagnosis of an inguinal hernia in the female includes
  A   a vaginal hydrocoele
  B   an encysted hydrocoele of the cord
  C   an hydrocoele in the canal of Nuck
  D   a femoral hernia
  E   Bartholin's cyst

807. In a strangulated inguinal hernia
  A   the constricting agent in children is the external abdominal ring
  B   omentum may be strangulated
  C   the large intestine is often involved
  D   irreducibility of the hernia is the pathognomonic physical sign
  E   reduction-en-masse resolves the problem satisfactorily

808. The patient with a Richter's hernia
  A   has, in fact, a sliding hernia
  B   has a hernia containing bladder within the wall of the sac
  C   has a Meckel's diverticulum within the sac
  D   should be treated by masterly inactivity
  E   is suitable for a truss

809. Regarding the union of fractures:
  A   Some fractures will unite in less than 3 weeks
  B   Spiral fractures take longer to unite than transverse fractures
  C   An oblique fracture of the shaft of the humerus in a child takes 3 weeks to unite
  D   Lower limb fractures take twice as long as upper limb fractures to unite
  E   Fractures in adults take twice as long to unite as fractures in children

810. The causes of non-union of a fracture include
  A   very slight bending movements during the healing phase
  B   infection of the fracture haematoma
  C   anoxia
  D   uraemia
  E   Paget's disease

811. **Regarding plaster of Paris splinting:**
    A After reduction of a fracture the plaster should be applied directly to and fashioned to the contours of the limb, allowed to set and then re-examined one week later
    B Patients should be given written instructions to report to hospital at the next fracture clinic if the limb distal to the fracture is painful and movement of muscles is impossible
    C If the limb is painful and movement is impossible the patient should be given analgesics and sedatives for relief and told to come back the next day
    D A first plaster on a fresh fracture should either not completely encircle the limb or it should be split
    E A first plaster should be padded and afterwards the limb is elevated

812. **A sarcoma usually spreads by**
    A seeding
    B lymphatic permeation
    C venous permeation
    D venous embolism
    E local extension

813. **In the clinical staging of carcinoma of the breast by the TNM classification, a staging of $T_2N_2M_1$ means**
    A tumour is more than 5 cm in diameter
    B skin is tethered to the tumour
    C axillary nodes are palpable but movable
    D there is oedema of the arm
    E there are no metastases

814. **Regarding the treatment of a clinically malignant parotid tumour:**
    A The tumour is usually radiosensitive
    B If operation is advised the facial nerve should be preserved
    C A frozen section during operation is helpful before any irrevocable mutilating step is taken
    D Excision of the mandible may be necessary
    E The prognosis is good

815. **Included in Sjogren's syndrome are**
    A dry eyes
    B rheumatoid arthritis
    C psoriasis
    D proptosis
    E dry mouth

816. If a patient has a branchial fistula
- A the external orifice is situated in the lower one-third of the neck near the posterior border of the sternomastoid
- B its discharges mucus
- C if complete, the internal opening is situated in the posterior pillar of the fauces behind the tonsil
- D it has been present from birth
- E a cervical auricle may be present

817. A cystic hygroma
- A is a type of lymphangioma
- B can obstruct labour
- C is mainly in the anterior triangle of the neck
- D is partly compressible
- E is barely translucent

818. Injury to the radial nerve in the axilla
- A can be caused by a crutch
- B is followed by paralysis of the triceps
- C is followed by inability to flex the elbow
- D causes anaesthesia in the anatomical snuff box area
- E is followed by inability to supinate the forearm

819. Which of the following conditions present as an 'acute red eye'?
- A Uveitis
- B Retinoblastoma
- C Acute glaucoma
- D Corneal ulceration
- E Amaurosis fugax

820. Perforation of the hard palate may be caused by
- A syphilis
- B friction of a malfitting dental plate
- C a palatal antrostomy
- D carcinoma of the tongue
- E bursting of an empyema through the floor of the antrum

821. When a casualty has severe injuries to the face:
- A The patient should be transported supine in an ambulance
- B An immediate danger to life is blood loss
- C If there is shock there may be other injuries
- D An immediate danger is respiratory obstruction due to inhaled blood
- E If there is bilateral fracture of the jaw the tongue may fall back

822. **Encysted hydrocoele of the cord**
    A is liable to be mistaken for a reducible inguinal hernia
    B moves downwards on traction of the testicle
    C is called a cyst of the canal of Nuck if situated within the inguinal canal and lateral to the spermatic cord
    D is a type of hydrocoele *en* Bisac
    E is a congenital hydrocoele

823. **Regarding the treatment of an hydrocoele:**
    A It may be tapped by a trocar
    B Tapping nearly always results in a cure
    C An haematocoele may follow tapping
    D Lord's operation of ruffing the tunica at the edge of the testis is a suitable procedure
    E Presents few problems post-operatively

824. **In the management of what one thinks is acute epididymo-orchitis one must be aware that**
    A the swelling may really be neoplastic
    B the scrotal skin may become adherent and the epididymis may discharge
    C the swelling may be due to tuberculosis
    D bed rest is unnecessary
    E the urine should be made acid

825. **A patient with a para-umbilical hernia**
    A has had it since infancy
    B often has adherent omentum in the sac
    C is usually a female
    D is unlikely to have a strangulated hernia
    E is often troubled by intertrigo

826. **Regarding an epigastric hernia:**
    A It is an hernia through the linea semilunaris
    B It commences as an extrusion of extraperitoneal fat
    C Normally it has a sac containing small intestine
    D The pain which the patient is suffering from may be due to a peptic ulcer
    E It requires the Mayo operation

827. **Regarding congenital abnormalities of the kidney:**
   A In horseshoe kidney a urogram shows that the lowest calyx on each side is reversed
   B Patients with congenital cystic kidneys tend to pass small amounts of concentrated urine
   C Congenital cystic kidneys may present with uraemia
   D A solitary renal cyst is not always congenital
   E Aberrent renal vessels accentuate an hydronephrosis

828. **Regarding congenital abnormalities of the ureter and renal pelvis:**
   A Duplication of a renal pelvis is the most common congenital abnormality of the upper renal tract
   B A double ureter is a cause of incontinence in the female
   C Megaureter occurs in infants with megacolon
   D Rarely the right ureter passes behind the inferior vena cava
   E An ureterocoele is prolapse of the ureter into the bladder

829. **Regarding a fracture of the medial epicondyle of the humerus:**
   A It is an avulsion injury
   B The fragment of bone may be rotated
   C The fragment of bone fortunately does not enter the elbow joint
   D A rotated fragment requires operative re-attachment to the epicondyle
   E Active and passive movements of the elbow joint should begin as soon as possible

830. **In dislocation of the shoulder**
   A the injury is produced by a fall with the arm fully abducted
   B the commonest position for the head of the humerus to move into is subspinous
   C the axillary nerve (circumflex) may be damaged
   D Kocher's method of reduction is no longer necessary
   E the easiest method of reduction is by simple pressure if a carefully administered general anaesthetic with a short acting muscle relaxant is given

831. Concerning fractures of the proximal humerus:
A The injury is through the anatomical neck following a fall on the outstretched hand
B Fracture of the surgical neck is common in the elderly
C Fracture of the anatomical neck may be combined with anterior dislocation of the shoulder
D Fracture of the surgical neck is treated by excision of the head of the humerus and replacement by a prosthesis
E Fracture of the anatomical neck with dislocation of the shoulder is best treated by rest in a sling with active mobilisation once pain has subsided

832. Regarding ulcerative colitis:
A It is linked with emotional stress
B It is best managed by prolonged cortisone therapy
C It is complicated by skin lesions
D If surgery is required, ileostomy is the treatment of choice
E The ileostomy opening should be in the midline just below the umbilicus

833. Regarding Crohn's disease:
A A perianal abscess or a fistula-in-ano is more likely to be associated with ulcerative colitis than Crohn's disease
B Steatorrhoea is uncommon in Crohn's disease
C Crohn's disease of the ileum is a cause of gallstone formation
D If Crohn's disease of the ileum is found at operation for a mistaken diagnosis of appendicitis, it is unwise to remove the appendix
E If the ileum is diseased and obstructed it is best to perform a primary resection

834. Concerning tumours of the small intestine:
A A leiomyoma can cause an intussusception
B In small intestinal polyposis pigmentation of the lips is the *sine qua non* of Peutz-Jegher's syndrome
C Lymphosarcoma of the small intestine runs a rapid course and is untreatable
D Adenocarcinoma does not occur in the jejunum
E A carcinoid tumour of the lower ileum should be resected by a right hemicolectomy

835. **A milk fistula**
    A occurs in lactating women
    B emanates from accessory nipples
    C is related to recurrent abscesses of the areolar region
    D can be related to duct ectasia
    E must be treated in the same way as a low fistula-in-ano

836. **Regarding tuberculosis of the breast:**
    A it is never seen today
    B it gets to the breast by retrograde lymphatic spread
    C it tends to occur in nullipara
    D sinuses with bluish edges are a feature
    E mastectomy is indicated

837. **The difference between eczema and Paget's disease of the nipple is that eczema**
    A is unilateral
    B is related to lactation
    C manifests vesicles
    D does not respond to simple treatment
    E is associated with a minute duct carcinoma within the breast

838. **In the operation of radical mastectomy (Halsted's operation)**
    A an area of skin 4–6 inches in diameter is removed
    B the nipple can be retained or transplanted to a new site
    C the latissimus dorsi is removed
    D the pectoralis muscle is retained
    E the long thoracic nerve should be spared

839. **According to the type, tuberculous peritonitis**
    A can be confused with peritoneal carcinomatosis
    B cause congenital hydrocoeles to appear
    C can be confused with an ovarian cyst
    D if causing obstruction should be treated by anastomosis between an obviously dilated loop and a collapsed loop of intestine
    E can present as a cold abscess near the umbilicus

840. **Regarding a wound of the mesentery of the small intestine:**
 A It causes pneumoperitoneum
 B It is commonly associated with rupture of the intestine
 C If the tear is transverse the wound is treated electively by suturing the tear
 D It should be suspected if there is bruising of the abdominal wall following a car accident even if seat belts are worn
 E It requires exteriorisation of the affected coil of intestine

841. **Regarding the blind loop syndrome:**
 A Its effects are due to bacterial fouling of the intestinal pathway
 B A high loop tends to produce anaemia
 C A low loop tends to produce steatorrhoea
 D Cure follows the prolonged use of antibiotics
 E A gastrocolic fistula behaves as a blind loop syndrome

842. **Incontinence may be**
 A nocturnal enuresis
 B total
 C due to the presence of an ureteric fistula
 D due to an aberrent ureter opening into the vagina in females
 E due to prostatectomy

843. **In a patient with a vesical calculus**
 A nocturnal frequency is a presenting symptom
 B pain is referred to the tip of the penis at the end of micturition
 C haematuria occurs at the beginning of micturition
 D there is more than a 90% chance that the stone can be demonstrated on an x-ray film
 E both litholapaxy and lithotomy are methods of treatment

844. **In malignant villous tumours of the bladder:**
 A The villi are elongated like a sea anemone
 B The growth tends to be well pedunculated
 C The growth may ulcerate
 D The growth may become encrusted with urinary salts
 E If two tumours are present it is a sure sign of malignancy

845. Regarding the biochemical effects of ureterocolic anastomosis:
A It results in reflux of colon contents up into the renal pelvis
B Loss of potassium occurs
C Alkalosis is typical
D The patient should take added salt in the diet
E Conversion to an ileal conduit should be considered

846. A patient with idiopathic thrombocytopaenia purpura
A is more likely to get purpuric lesions in the dependent areas
B usually has a very large spleen
C tends to respond to steroid therapy
D is rarely helped in the control of the bleeding tendency by splenectomy
E often has the bleeding tendency aggravated by massive and rapid transfusions

847. Regarding the stages in the elective removal of the spleen:
A A Morris incision is made
B The first step is to pass a hand round the outer surface of the spleen to avulse adhesions and to divide the posterior layer of the lienorenal ligament
C The lesser sac between stomach, colon and spleen is well opened to give access to the splenic vessels
D Splenunculi should be looked for
E The wound should not be drained if haemostasis appears to be satisfactory

848. Regarding rupture of the liver:
A Rupture of the left lobe is more common than the right lobe because the right lobe is more solid
B Packing of the liver is to be avoided
C Major hepatic resection may be necessary
D The abdominal cavity need not be drained
E Haemobilia is a complication

849. An amoebic liver abscess
A is a termination of amoebic hepatitis
B is due to entamoeba coli
C is multiple in 70% of cases
D is insidious in the presentation of clinical features
E is not excluded if the amoebae are not found in the stools

850. **In the management of fracture of the mandible:**
    A The simplest method is to wire the jaws together in occlusion by interdental wiring
    B Infection is unusual because the blood supply to the head is extensive
    C In edentulous patients either dentures or acrylic moulds are wired to the alveolus and thence together
    D A light diet is given
    E Aspiration pneumonia is unlikely

851. **If a patient aged 50 has osteomyelitis of the jaw**
    A an injudicious tooth extraction may have been performed under local anaesthetic
    B the mandible is less affected than the maxilla because it has a better blood supply
    C an early x-ray will confirm the diagnosis
    D operation is necessary to relieve tension
    E bone recovery is poor

852. **The fibro-osseous group of jaw tumours include**
    A ivory osteoma
    B Paget's disease
    C leontiasis ossea
    D monostotic fibrous dysplasia
    E myeloid epulis

853. **Regarding carcinoma of the pancreas:**
    A 70% of the patients have a periampullary carcinoma
    B It is usually a medullary carcinoma
    C If occurring in the body and tail it tends to involve the duodenojejunal junction
    D Troisier's sign is commonly positive
    E The patient may present with copious watery bright green vomit

854. **Regarding a pelvic abscess:**
    A Pus can accumulate without serious constitutional disturbance
    B Constipation is a characteristic symptom
    C On rectal examination the abscess feels like a hard apple
    D The abscess may discharge spontaneously through the rectum
    E In the case of a large abscess drainage should be by means of a low abdominal laparotomy

855. In a patient with a subphrenic abscess
- A there is loss of weight
- B there can be a pleural effusion
- C there is a relative but not absolute leucocytosis
- D a diagnostic needling through the ninth intercostal space is performed prior to exposure of a posterior supradiaphragmatic abscess
- E a small drainage tube should be left in after opening the abscess

856. Regarding paralysis of muscles and their management:
- A The paralysed muscle becomes shorter than its non-paralysed fellow
- B A totally paralysed limb has a strong tendency to deform
- C Full joint movements are maintained by daily passive movement
- D Splintage helps to prevent deformity
- E In a child it often becomes necessary to lengthen tendons of unopposed muscles acting on the joint

857. Regarding pes cavus:
- A The instep is high with flattening and splaying of the toes
- B The deformity seems to be caused by weakness of the intrinsic muscles of the foot
- C Another factor causing the deformity is the presence of a Dupuytren's contracture of the plantar fascia
- D In childhood the foot is painful and the contracted plantar fascia is tender
- E Friedreich's ataxia should be excluded

858. Associated with hallux valgus are included
- A an overriding of the second toe by the first
- B an underriding of the second toe by the first
- C rheumatoid arthritis of the first metatarsophalangeal joint
- D an inflamed adventitious bursa
- E an exostosis on the lateral side of the head of the first metatarsal

859. Retrosternal goitre
- A usually arises from ectopic thyroid tissue
- B can be of the plunging type
- C can cause a 'scabbard' trachea
- D is treated in the first instance by radio-iodine
- E may have to be removed piecemeal

860. **In Wayne's clinical diagnostic index of thyrotoxicosis (+ or − values given to symptoms):**
    A   Increased appetite scores −3
    B   Decreased weight scores +3
    C   A preference for heat scores −5
    D   Hyperkinetic movements score −1
    E   Atrial fibrillation scores +1

861. **Pretibial myxoedema**
    A   is a thickening of the skin by a mucin-like deposit
    B   may be cyanotic when cold
    C   is an occasional feature of myxoedema
    D   is associated with low levels of L.A.T.S.
    E   may be associated with clubbing of the fingers and toes

862. **In the choice of a therapeutic agent for the treatment of thyrotoxicosis, which of the following are acceptable?**
    A   For a diffuse toxic goitre under 45 – radio-iodine
    B   For a toxic nodular goitre – radio-iodine
    C   For a toxic nodule – surgery
    D   For recurrent thyrotoxicosis after adequate surgery over 45 – radio-iodine
    E   For failure of previous treatment with antithyroid drugs or radio-iodine – surgery

863. **Strictures of the common bile duct**
    A   are usually due to operative trauma
    B   are related to ignorance of the anatomical anomalies of the bile ducts
    C   can be due to sclerosing cholangitis
    D   present immediately after operation with jaundice
    E   can be repaired over a T-tube

864. **A choledochoduodenostomy**
    A   is an operation which is followed by much post-operative morbidity
    B   is used in the treatment of choledochal cyst
    C   is used for malignant obstruction due to carcinoma of the gall bladder
    D   can be used in an elderly patient with an unresolved problem at the lower end of the bile duct
    E   must not be performed if the common bile duct is less than 1 cm diameter and if the stoma is going to be less than 2 cm

865. **Regarding biliary fistula:**
   A They are always external
   B External fistulae cause little biochemical disturbance
   C They tend to dry up in the passage of time
   D A patient can vomit gallstones as a result of a particular fistula
   E Stones can be extruded through the umbilicus

866. **Regarding Perthe's disease of the head of the femur:**
   A Girls are more commonly affected than boys
   B The condition presents with a limp
   C The younger the child the worse the prognosis
   D If the femoral head becomes deformed osteoarthrosis may occur in adult life
   E The most effective way of reducing the chances of a deformed head of femur is to confine the child to bed for 2–3 years

867. **In supraspinatus tendonitis**
   A the tendon may degenerate and rupture
   B the patient is likely to have nonspecific urethritis
   C the patient has the painful arc syndrome
   D a frozen shoulder may occur
   E the condition is permanent and requires frequent manipulation of the shoulder

868. **Regarding the carpal tunnel syndrome:**
   A the patient may have rheumatoid arthritis
   B the patient may have myxoedema
   C pain in the hand occurs at night when the arm falls down outside the bed
   D weakness of the muscles supplied by the ulnar nerve is likely to occur
   E an operation opening up the tendon sheaths is indicated

869. **In tuberculous lymphadenitis of the neck**
   A the nodes usually are discrete
   B sinuses can occur
   C removal of the affected nodes help the patient to overcome the disease elsewhere in the body
   D the key to resection is to identify and dissect the nodes away from the internal jugular vein
   E the spinal accessory nerve should be spared

870. **When clinically malignant lymph nodes appear in the neck**
   A the site of the primary is easy to find
   B the testis could be the primary site
   C palpable cervical lymph nodes draining a primary tumour are not necessarily involved by growth
   D adherence of a node or tumour to the mandible is a contraindication to surgery
   E when the cervical lymph nodes are fixed it is helpful to make an incision directly over them to obtain a biopsy

871. **In classical block dissection of the neck**
   A the sternomastoid is detached from its lower attachment and resutured at the end of the operation
   B a length of the internal jugular vein is removed
   C the common carotid artery is tied
   D the contents of the submental triangle are removed
   E the cervical branch of the facial nerve is severed

872. **Simple goitre**
   A is due to stimulation of the thyroid gland by the anterior pituitary
   B may occur in lowland areas
   C may be due to enzyme deficiency within the thyroid gland
   D may be caused by excessive iodide intake
   E is referred to on the Continent as 'struma'.

873. **In rupture of the bulbous urethra:**
   A Retention of urine is one of the signs
   B The patient should be encouraged to pass urine
   C If he cannot pass urine the patient should be catheterised on the spot
   D The urethra should be completely repaired by sutures
   E The perineal wound, if an operation is performed, is packed not stitched

874. **The complications of urethral stricture include**
   A Dupuytren's contracture
   B hydronephrosis
   C periurethral abscess
   D hernia
   E Peyronie's disease

875. Granuloma inguinale
- A is synonymous with lymphogranuloma venereum
- B is caused by a virus
- C causes an ulcer in the groin
- D is complicated by Peyronie's disease
- E is treated by oxytetracycline

876. Incomplete descent of the testis
- A is arrest of the testis in some part of its path to the scrotum
- B occurs in 30% of premature infants
- C does not affect the internal secretory activity of the testis
- D is commonest on the left side
- E is present if the testis on traction cannot be made to touch the bottom of the scrotum

877. Concerning tuberculosis of bones and joints:
- A The primary focus may be in the gastrointestinal tract
- B The condition is always due to the human strain of *mycobacterium tuberculosis*
- C The disease starts in bone and not synovial membrane
- D Following destruction of bone a joint may dislocate
- E A bony ankylosis is the final outcome if it is treated satisfactorily

878. Action in the preparation of a patient for thyroidectomy for thyrotoxicosis includes:
- A The patient should be brought into an euthyroid state
- B Recording changes in weight and sleeping pulse rate
- C The use of chlorpropamide for preparation
- D The use of potassium perchlorate and Lugol's iodine (or potassium iodide)
- E Propranolol which does not act on the thyroid itself and has to be carried on post-operatively

879. Concerning cystin calculi:
- A They are wont to appear in the urinary tract of patients with cystinuria
- B Cystinuria is an inborn error of metabolism
- C Cystin crystals are hexagonal
- D They are radio-opaque owing to the calcium they contain
- E The stones are soft, like beeswax, often yellow and change on exposure to a greenish hue

880. Regarding the histological appearance of leukoplakia:
- A An acanthosis occurs
- B The rete pegs are prolonged and widened
- C Epithelial pearls are not seen
- D The basal cells are like those in Paget's disease of the nipple
- E Carcinoma *in situ* may be present

881. In tuberculous tenosynovitis
- A the endothelial lining of the tendon sheath may contain miliary tubercles
- B very little free fluid may be present
- C an effusion containing 'melon-seed' bodies may occur
- D the term 'compound palmar ganglion' is used
- E treatment may include dissection and removal of the tendon sheath

882. Osteoarthritis
- A is osteoarthrosis which is the same as osteoarthritis
- B is primarily due to abrasion caused by a breakdown in joint lubrication
- C is manifested in the first place by fibrillation of articular cartilage
- D causes fibrosis of the capsule of a joint
- E causes the appearance of bone 'cysts' in cancellous bone adjacent to a joint

883. Signs of ascites may be due to
- A Meigs' syndrome
- B endometriosis
- C pseudomyxoma peritoneii
- D Pick's disease
- E Arnold-Chiari malformation

884. An upper brachial plexus injury:
- A Is known as a Klumpke paralysis
- B Affects only infants
- C The fifth cervical root is always involved
- D Sensory changes are absent if the fifth root only is involved
- E The forearm hangs in the pronated position

885. **The clinical situations which are most likely to cause death in the terminal stages of carcinoma of the tongue include**
   A haemorrhage
   B bronchopneumonia
   C malnutrition
   D distant metastases
   E oedema of the glottis

886. **Rheumatoid arthritis**
   A can occur in childhood
   B runs a more benign course in the young than in the elderly
   C is progressive and relentless without remission
   D is associated with muscle wasting
   E reveals large osteophytes in sclerotic bone adjacent to the joint

887. **If a female patient complains of a discharge from the nipple:**
   A If a lump in the breast is present, remove the lump
   B If it is localised to one duct a microdochectomy is indicated
   C If discharge from more than one duct gives a positive result to the haemoglobin test and the patient is over 40, a simple mastectomy is advised
   D If the discharge gives a negative haemoglobin result the patient is re-examined at intervals and the occult blood test is repeated
   E If a lump appears, remove the lump

888. **A Warthin's tumour is**
   A a carcinoma of the submandibular salivary gland
   B a malignant change in a brachial cyst
   C contains eosinophilic epithelium and cysts
   D an adenolymphoma
   E usually a swelling towards the lower pole of the parotid

889. **Ankylosing spondylitis**
   A can be regarded as a variant of rheumatoid arthritis
   B is a process of calcification and ossification of cartilage
   C is most common in women
   D can be partly diagnosed by tissue typing
   E tends to begin in the sacroiliac joints

890. **In the case of unilateral congenital dislocation of the hip in children between six months and seven years:**
    A Reduction should be effected and maintained
    B The older the child the more difficult the reduction becomes
    C Maintenance of reduction may be difficult because the acetabulum is abnormally shallow and vertical
    D Open reduction should always be performed
    E The results of treatment are worse than the disease itself

891. **Regarding club foot:**
    A If the foot is fixed in dorsiflexion the deformity is called 'equinus'
    B If the foot is inverted and adducted the deformity is called 'valgus'
    C The most common deformity is 'talipes equinovarus'
    D The condition should be diagnosed when the infant is between 1–2 years old
    E Most cases can be treated satisfactorily by manipulation and splintage if it is started early enough

892. **Fournier's gangrene of the scrotum is related to**
    A aortic bifurcation embolus
    B infection
    C minor injuries
    D no obvious cause
    E filariasis

893. **Concerning rejection after kidney transplantation:**
    A All allotransplants have some degree of rejection
    B Anuria means acute tubular necrosis and failure of the transplant
    C Hyperacute rejection may occur within minutes of the operation
    D The kidney becomes swollen but because it is a transplant it is not tender
    E External radiation may be indicated to reverse rejection

894. **If the circumflex (axillary nerve) is cut**
    A the deltoid muscle is paralysed
    B the triceps is paralysed
    C the teres minor is paralysed
    D there is a patch of anaesthesia over the acromion process
    E the pectoralis minor muscle is paralysed

895. Regarding carcinoma of the tongue:
- A Ankyloglossia occurs when a carcinoma begins on the dorsum of the tongue
- B It may simply present with a lump in the neck
- C Alteration of the voice is an early feature of carcinoma of the back of the tongue
- D A carcinoma which begins on one side of the anterior two-thirds of the tongue soon spreads across the midline to the other side
- E In many instances the lymphatics draining the anterior two-thirds of the tongue and the floor of the mouth transverse the periosteum of the mandible

896. In Cushing's disease the results of the investigations include
- A a fasting eosinophil count over 30 per ml is good evidence of the condition
- B the basal metabolic rate is raised
- C the insulin tolerance test reveals a resistance to the action of insulin
- D there is a strong positive calcium balance
- E x-ray of the skeleton show osteopetrosis

897. Duct ectasia of the breast
- A occurs in young multipara
- B means that the ducts are dilated with mucus
- C presents with a worm-like swelling extending radially from the nipple
- D is associated with periductal inflammation with lymphocytes and plasma cells
- E is a premalignant condition

898. The right recurrent laryngeal nerve may be damaged by
- A malignant infiltration of the thyroid gland
- B operation on the thyroid gland
- C operation on a patent ductus arteriosus
- D secondary lymph nodes from carcinoma of the bronchus
- E pressure by an aneurysm of the aortic arch

899. In extracapsular fracture of the proximal femur
 A external rotation and shortening of the leg occurs
 B traction and bed rest is suitable treatment for the elderly patient for three months
 C treatment by traction and rest is not acceptable in the treatment of young adults
 D simple nailing (such as the Smith Petersen nail) is the most suitable treatment
 E avascular necrosis of the head is almost unknown

900. The immediate postoperative complications of thyroidectomy include
 A secondary haemorrhage
 B laryngeal oedema
 C hypothyroidism
 D keloid scarring
 E surgical emphysema

901. In the management of gallstone colic
 A pethidine (demerol) alone causes spasm of the sphincter of Oddi
 B the use of suitably covered hot water bottle and heating pads to the right hypochondrium is outmoded
 C one of the hyocyamus group of drugs should precede the giving of proper doses of morphine or pethidine
 D the use of pethidine (demerol) does not conflict with the use of other drugs the patient may be having
 E emergency cholecystectomy is a good way of solving the patient's problem

902. Fractures of the patella
 A can be caused by indirect violence
 B are stellate in appearance if caused by indirect violence
 C if stellate are treated by circumferential wiring
 D if transverse are best treated by patellectomy
 E are never vertical fractures

903. The indications for choledochotomy following cholecystectomy include
 A small stones in the gall bladder and cystic duct
 B a dilated cystic duct
 C a dilated thick-walled common bile duct
 D an attack of gallstone ileus
 E a stone impacted in Hartmann's pouch

904. Total thyroidectomy
A is indicated for papillary carcinoma
B is indicated for medullary carcinoma
C is often impossible for anaplastic carcinoma
D includes the removal of all the parathyroid glands as there is usually an ectopic gland in the mediastinum
E necessarily means the division of both recurrent laryngeal nerves

905. In patients with a fractured shaft of femur
A blood loss of a litre is easily concealed
B fixed traction using the Thomas splint is one method of treatment
C traction methods require constant attention
D stiffness of the knee is a common complication
E after union 2 cm of shortening is acceptable

906. In the management of carcinoma of the tongue
A the Wasserman or similar reactions should be known
B dental sepsis is treated
C small lesions are excised by wide excisional biopsy
D sub-total glossectomy is indicated in large lesions which do not respond to radiotherapy
E diathermy excision is the best technique for the removal of tumours

907. In patients with papillary carcinoma of the thyroid
A the growth is usually single and localised
B after operation TSH production should be suppressed by full doses of thyroxin
C there is a high incidence of lymph node metastases
D block dissection of the neck is necessary
E the prognosis is poor

908. For cholecystectomy
A a right paramedian incision can be used
B a large tightly distended gall bladder should be aspirated
C cholecystectomy forceps are applied to the cystic duct
D the cystic artery is clamped with long artery forceps
E a drain is unnecessary after a straightforward removal

909. **Regarding radiotherapy for carcinoma of the tongue:**
    A Radioactive needles are no longer used
    B A radioactive isotope is used
    C It is a useful treatment of lymphatic metastases
    D A growth involving the jaw should be excised and not irradiated
    E Irradiation improves the five year survival rate to 40%

910. **Regarding pleomoprhic salivary adenomas:**
    A Of the salivary neoplasms that arise in the parotid 45% are benign pleomorphic adenomas
    B Malignant change does not occur
    C The arrangement of cells includes strands, duct like formation or in sheets
    D A mucoid material is produced
    E The benign pleomorphic adenoma cells tend to penetrate the thin capsule into the surrounding gland

911. **The extensor apparatus of the knee includes**
    A the patella
    B the ligamentum patellae
    C the biceps femoris
    D the patella retinaculae
    E the popliteus

912. **If a patient has acute pyelonephritis**
    A the infection can be blood-borne to the kidney from a boil on the skin
    B the usual organism is the *proteus mirabilis*
    C in the presence of *Esch. coli* infection the urine is alkaline
    D it may present with sudden abdominal pain and vomiting
    E the differential diagnosis includes pneumonia and acute appendicitis

913. **In the investigation and assessment of a patient who may have an adenocarcinoma of the kidney:**
    A A patient with haematuria, pain and a palpable renal tumour is almost certain to have metastases
    B All patients with haematuria should wait for cystoscopy as soon as bleeding has ceased
    C Excretory pyelography is always conclusive
    D Retrograde pyelography may, if a tumour is present, show a characteristic failure of the contrast to enter a major calyx
    E Growths of the lower pole displace the ureter laterally

914. **Which of the following are consistent with a diagnosis of Hashimoto's disease?**
   A   A painful gland
   B   Hyperthyroidism
   C   Hypothyroidism
   D   Swelling localised to one lobe
   E   A high 48-hour PB^{131}I uptake test result in the absence of a previous thyroidectomy or radio-iodine therapy

915. **Regarding the angular and torsional deformities of the leg during growth:**
   A   Bow leg is more common than knock-knee
   B   In-toeing is more common than splay foot
   C   The degree of bow leg is measured by the distance between the medial malleoli
   D   Knock knee may be due to rickets
   E   Adjustments to footwear by wedging corrects the deformities

916. **Regarding idiopathic scoliosis:**
   A   It does not appear in infancy and early childhood
   B   Once advanced structural deformity has occurred it is irreversible
   C   Careful radiological supervision with accurate measurement of the curvature is essential in early management
   D   A Milwaukee brace may be successful as a non-operative method of preventing deterioration
   E   It is best to perform surgery well before skeletal maturity

917. **Senile osteoporosis**
   A   can only be detected radiologically when about 40% of the skeleton has been lost
   B   is manifest on x-ray of the spine as a 'fish head' appearance of the vertebral bodies
   C   causes a lot of bone pain
   D   causes delayed healing if a fracture occurs
   E   is, through progressive fatigue, a likely cause of fracture of the neck of the femur

918. **In complete ectopia vesicae**
   A   effluxes of urine from the ureteric orifices can be seen
   B   there is hypospadias
   C   umbilical hernia may be present
   D   the patient has a waddling gait
   E   the results of surgery are good

919. **In the operation for thyroglossal fistula**
    A the track is dissected as it passes behind the hyoid cartilage onwards up the tongue
    B the track is dissected as it passes behind, below and in front of the hyoid cartilage
    C the middle portion of the hyoid cartilage is excised
    D the track is dissected upwards until it enters the mouth close to the frenum of the tongue
    E the track is dissected and excised with a central core of lingual muscle extending centrally towards the foramen caecum

920. **The biochemical findings which support a diagnosis of hyperparathyroidism include**
    A diminution of the serum calcium
    B elevation of the serum phosphorus
    C elevation of the serum alkaline phosphatase
    D increased excretion of calcium in the urine
    E elevated serum T4

921. **In Reiter's disease**
    A conjunctivitis occurs
    B acute hydrarthrosis is present
    C a urethral smear reveals streptococci
    D there is keratoderma blenorrhagicum of the heel
    E a urethral smear reveals gonococci

922. **Regarding carcinoma of the head of the pancreas:**
    A Biopsy is limited by safety considerations and histological dubieties
    B A periampillary growth is more suitable than a growth of the head proper for an attempt at cure
    C Pancreaticoduodenotomy gives a better 5-year survival rate than a palliative operation for a growth of the head proper
    D Total pancreatectomy must be performed
    E Cholecystojejunotomy is indicated as a palliative operation

923. **In Riedel's thyroditis**
    A the thyroid tissue is replaced by fibrous tissue
    B the swelling is soft and bulky
    C a scan shows no uptake over the swelling
    D an anaplastic carcinoma is in fact present
    E there may be mediastinal fibrosis

924. **The desirable treatments of benign enlargement of the prostate include**
    A   a permanent suprapubic catheter
    B   preliminary vasectomy
    C   a transvesical prostatectomy
    D   division of the external sphincter
    E   perurethral resection

925. **The diagnostic features in the first three days of acute pancreatitis include**
    A   agonising pain localised to the epigastrium
    B   vomiting and retching
    C   shock
    D   a tender palpable mass in the epigastrium
    E   glycosuria

926. **In acute maxillary sinusitis with acute empyema of the antrum**
    A   one of the causes may be a periodontal abscess
    B   an x-ray shows an opaque antrum
    C   a flow of pus can be obtained when the head is held upwards and backwards
    D   a diagnostic proof puncture of the antrum is performed through the nose
    E   a Caldwell-Luc operation is necessary in order to achieve resolution

927. **Chronic otitis media**
    A   necessarily follows an acute otitis
    B   presents with profuse otorrhoea
    C   causes marked conduction deafness
    D   may require a radical mastoidectomy
    E   is complicated by labyrinthitis

928. **An eighth nerve tumour**
    A   presents with bilateral deafness
    B   causes vertigo
    C   causes loss of the corneal reflex
    D   is treated by radiotherapy
    E   carries a poor prognosis

929. The treatment of acute retention due to carcinoma of the prostate include
- A an indwelling (Gibbon) catheter
- B 25 mg stilboestrol four times daily for two weeks
- C cystectomy
- D immediate retropubic prostatectomy
- E radiotherapy

930. Regarding a hydatid cyst:
- A The endocyst secretes the hydatid fluid and the laminated membrane
- B Within the brood capsules the scolices (heads of future worms) develop
- C The pseudocyst looks like a child's uncoloured balloon filled with water
- D Calcification means deterioration in the host
- E Effective treatment is surgical

931. Porta-systemic shunting of operations
- A should not be performed if the patient is significantly jaundiced
- B should not be performed if the patient's serum albumin is more than 30 g/l (3g/100 ml)
- C should be reserved for patients who are bleeding from varices
- D are avoided in the presence of ascites
- E are needed to prevent bleeding from oesophageal varices before it ever happens

932. Primary carcinoma of the liver
- A tends to occur in children and older people
- B causes a Pel-Ebstein type of fever
- C causes the CEA level in the plasma to be raised
- D cannot be diagnosed by CT scanning (even if available)
- E is associated with ascites in about 40% of patients at the time of first examination

933. Gallstones
- A may contain protein
- B may contain bacteria
- C are made of bile salts mixed with cholesterol
- D are best dissolved by giving the patient a long course of lithocholic acid
- E may be present in a patient who has acholuric jaundice

934. The following are consistent with a diagnosis of chronic prostatitis:
   A Referred pain down the legs
   B The seminal vesicles are infected
   C In the three glass test, prostatitis is present if threads are seen in the last glass
   D Examination of prostatic fluid is performed on a catheter specimen of urine
   E Urethroscopy reveals an enlarged oedematous verumontanum

935. In acute otitis media:
   A It is secondary to furunculosis of the ear
   B It presents with painful deaf ear
   C Antibiotics are helpful only if given early and as a full course
   D Myringotomy is performed when pus appears
   E Chronic otitis media is the usual complication

936. If a patient is believed to have acute pancreatitis
   A laparotomy is essential if there is any doubt about the diagnosis
   B morphine in the treatment of the pain should be used in conjunction with Pethidine (demerol or demerol hydrochloride)
   C intravenous fluids increase the oedema of the pancreas
   D gallstones are present in at least 30% of patients
   E a pseudocyst may occur later

937. Regarding peptic ulcers and malignancy:
   A A duodenal ulcer can undergo malignant change
   B A giant gastric ulcer is usually malignant
   C A gastric ulcer in the presence of achlorhydria is likely to be malignant
   D A gastric cancer at the edge of the ulcer separates the muscularis mucosae from the muscle layer
   E Epithelial proliferation and downgrowths at the edge of a gastric ulcer means malignancy

938. Regarding fistula-in-ano:
- A A high intersphincteric anal fistula runs between the internal and external sphincters along the plane of the longitudinal muscle fibres
- B A high intersphincteric fistula is treated by dividing the external sphincter
- C A high transphincteric fistula should be treated by laying the track open
- D A low level fistula will respond to and heal under the influence of antibiotics
- E A protective colostomy may be required in the treatment of a high level fistula

939. Severance of the radial nerve in the axilla causes
- A paralysis of the deltoid
- B inability to extend the elbow
- C complete inability to extend the fingers with the hand supported
- D inability to supinate the forearm
- E anaesthesia over the dorsum of the forearm and back of the hand or wrist

940. Severance of the sciatic nerve in the buttock above the origin of the hamstring causes
- A paralysis of the knee extensors
- B foot drop
- C loss of ankle jerk
- D sensory loss to the whole of the leg below the knee
- E trophic ulcers on the sole of the foot

941. Regarding miscellaneous conditions related to the supraorbital margin and the eyelids:
- A A Meibomian cyst is a sebaceous cyst of the eyelid
- B A hordeolum is a stye
- C A midline subcutaneous cyst which empties on pressure is a dermoid cyst
- D An external angular dermoid should be x-rayed before removal
- E A mucocoele of the lachrymal sac causes a swelling in the outer canthus of the eye

942. **True cysts of the pancreas**
    A   are more common than pseudocysts
    B   may present as a solid swelling
    C   may be attributed to the *taenia echinococcus*
    D   if in the head, are treated by pancreatico-duodenectomy (Whipple's operation)
    E   if in the body, are suitable for cystogastrostomy

943. **Regarding prolapsed intervertebral disc:**
    A   In some 20% of cases there is no history of injury
    B   About 20% of prolapsed discs occur in the cervical region at the C5/6 and C6/7 levels
    C   Narrowing of the intervertebral joint is characteristic of all cases of prolapsed disc
    D   Massive protrusions may occur as the result of major cervical injuries
    E   The spinal canal is narrowed by the formation of a Schmorl's node

944. **Regarding seventh nerve palsy:**
    A   An infranuclear lesion involves only the lower half of the face
    B   It can be caused by middle ear disease
    C   All types of extracranial palsy are called Bell's palsy
    D   It is an indication of malignancy when associated with a parotid tumour
    E   Corneal ulceration may occur

945. **In the management of wounds where peripheral nerves have been severed**
    A   primary nerve suture should not be performed
    B   nerve suture should be postponed until three months after the injury
    C   delayed nerve suture is more difficult than primary nerve suture because of the epineural fibrosis
    D   at the primary debridement the area should be explored to identify other nerves in the vicinity
    E   the quality of regeneration is less perfect after neurotmesis than after axonotmesis

946. **The objectives of operations for peptic ulcers are**
    A to end with a situation where the patient is always free from pain and complications if he keeps to an ulcer type of diet
    B in duodenal ulcer, to reduce the parietal cell mass or to reduce stimuli to acid secretion
    C in gastric ulcer, to aim at excision of the ulcer bearing area and the stomach proximal to the ulcer
    D to improve the emptying of the stomach
    E to avert the slight risk that gastric ulcers become malignant in time

947. **Regarding an anastomotic ulcer following operations for duodenal ulcer:**
    A It is most likely to occur after a polya gastrectomy
    B It is usually in the mesenteric side of the jejunum
    C A piece of suture material from the previous operation is frequently found in its base
    D The pain it causes is usually felt in the right hypochondrium and travels down the right side of the abdomen
    E The pain is not relieved by antacids or milk

948. **Regarding malignant tumours of the anus:**
    A Most of the tumours are papillary columnar cell carcinomas
    B Primary lymph drainage is to the inferior mesenteric nodes
    C Anal cancer can masquerade as an anal fissure
    D Small squamous cell lesions can be treated by wide local excision
    E Basaloid tumours should be treated by radiotherapy

949. **Post-operative synergistic gangrene**
    A is a complication of appendicitis
    B is a complication of drainage of an empyema thoracis
    C begins in the muscle layers
    D is a self-localising condition
    E requires hyperbaric oxygen therapy, if available

950. **Concerning congenital problems causing acute intestinal obstruction in the newborn:**
    A Atresia and stenosis of the duodenum occur with about equal frequency
    B Supraduodenal atresia is distinguished from oesophageal atresia by the fact that there is no dribbling of saliva
    C Meconium ileus is due to ileal atresia
    D Volvulus of the midgut includes the caecum
    E Atresia of the ileum may present as a perforation

951. **Patients who have an hiatus hernia**
    A usually have a rolling hernia
    B may be infants
    C can be thin
    D may develop pneumonitis
    E are best treated by surgery

952. **Regarding volvulus of the intestinal tract:**
    A It occurs in newborn Africans
    B It is related to eating diets which are deficient in roughage
    C It is common in Eastern Europe
    D The twisted loop is mainly full of faeces
    E Decompression by the use of a trochar and wide bore cannuli is necessary before laparotomy to untwist the bowel

953. **Bolus obstruction**
    A can follow eating unripe apples
    B is a problem after partial gastrectomy
    C can be caused by a gallstone
    D is treated by enemas
    E should be investigated by an emergency barium meal

954. **Non-malignant strictures of the rectum include those which are**
    A a spasmodic variety with fibrosis of the external sphincter due to anal fissure
    B post-operative after haemorrhoidectomy
    C due to endometriosis
    D due to granuloma venereum
    E congenital in origin

955. **Among the disposing factors causing postoperative complications are included**
    A lack of analgesics
    B a many-tailed bandage of the abdomen
    C the necessary use of endotracheal tubes
    D dehydration
    E the menopause

956. **Regarding traumatic diaphragmatic hernia:**
    A The diaphragm can be ruptured without an external wound
    B In crush injuries the dome is usually torn
    C A hernia of intestines into the chest follows
    D There is a large hernial sac which becomes adherent to the lungs
    E Strangulation does not occur

957. **The clinical features of mitral stenosis include**
    A systemic embolism
    B haematemesis
    C ascites
    D high blood pressure
    E warm vasodilated extremities

958. **In the management of a patient with a spinal cord injury**
    A the patient should be turned every six hours
    B plaster immobilisation increases the risk of pressure sores
    C meteorism should be allowed to occur
    D passive movements of the limbs are necessary
    E operations such as plating are indicated to relieve existing damage to the cord

959. **If a patient has had a vagotomy for a duodenal ulcer**
    A he is often troubled by obstinate constipation
    B he tends to get 'blown up' with wind
    C a gastric ulcer may occur
    D he tends to suffer from calcium deficiency
    E he is very likely to suffer from a 'bolus obstruction'.

960. **Regarding a leather bottle stomach:**
    A There is a proliferation of fibrous tissue in the submucosa
    B The mucous membrane is indurated and hypertrophic
    C Lymph nodes tend not to be affected at an early stage
    D It can be confused with Crohn's disease of the stomach
    E Gastrectomy is likely to be curative

961. **Prolonged parenteral antibiotic therapy**
    A is necessary for subphrenic abscess
    B is necessary for ileocaecal actinomycosis
    C can cause intestinal obstruction if used for peritonitis
    D can mask the general signs of an intra-abdominal abscess
    E is *the* cause of staphylococcal enterocolitis

962. A patient with a true pilonidal sinus
- A has a post-anal dermoid
- B could well be a barber
- C has hair follicles in the walls of the sinus
- D has it within the fibres of the corrigator cutis ani
- E tends to get a fistula-in-ano as a result of secondary abscesses

963. Regarding tumours of the spinal canal:
- A dumb-bell tumours are extradural neurofibromas
- B neurofibromas may cause erosion of an intervertebral foramen
- C intradural tumours may be neurofibromas
- D extramedullary tumours account for 75% of intradural tumours
- E most intramedullary tumours occur in the lumbar part of the spinal cord

964. A female patient with pruritis ani
- A may have a fistula-in-ano
- B may have psoriasis
- C may have scabies
- D can be improved with podophyllin resin
- E should have the urine tested for the presence of sugar

965. Complete prolapse of the rectum
- A is common in children
- B is virtually an intussusception of the rectum upon itself, but there is no intussuscipiens
- C when large may contain a pouch of peritoneum containing small intestine
- D can be distinguished from rectosigmoid intussusception
- E is best excised

966. If a child is born with a myelocoele
- A gross talipes is obvious
- B meningitis is likely to occur
- C it contains only cerebrospinal fluid
- D an elliptical raw surface is seen
- E operation should be delayed for three months

967. A duodenal fistula
- A is a complication of trauma to the duodenum
- B is a complication of gastrostomy
- C may follow a right hemicolectomy
- D causes excoriation of the skin
- E requires immediate operation to prevent dehydration and hypoproteinaemia

968. Patients with acholuric familial jaundice
- A have a palpable spleen
- B are likely to have pure cholesterol gallstones
- C have a spleen which is at fault
- D require treatment by splenectomy
- E retain the tendency to haemolysis

969. Regarding secondary deposits in the spine:
- A They cause severe local pain
- B They cause girdle pain
- C A malignant parotid tumour does not give rise to bone secondaries
- D A hypernephroma normally gives rise to osteosclerotic secondaries
- E Laminectomy and bone grafting is used to treat vertebral collapse

970. Concerning operations for carcinoma of the large intestine:
- A Carcinoma of the caecum should be treated by caecectomy
- B Carcinoma of the hepatic flexure may involve the right ureter
- C Carcinoma of the transverse colon is best treated if the excision includes the hepatic and the splenic flexures
- D Carcinoma of the splenic flexure is best excised with four inches of transverse and descending colon (above and below)
- E Resection of the pelvic colon should include resection of the splenic flexure

971. Regarding colostomy:
- A It is a type of faecal fistula
- B The descending colon is suitable for a loop colostomy
- C Closure of a temporary colostomy is best performed by an intraperitoneal closure
- D A terminal colostomy is best sited in the right iliac fossa
- E If the 'lateral space' is not closed small bowel obstruction and strangulation is a likely complication

972. **Regarding intestinal obstruction with strangulation:**
    A   Mesenteric vascular occlusion due to an embolus is not a form of strangulation
    B   The loss of circulating blood volume due to strangulation of several feet of small intestine is considerable
    C   When obstruction occurs distension of the proximal intestine begins forthwith
    D   There is more toxic absorption into the circulation from strangulation in an external hernia than an internal strangulation
    E   In closed loop obstruction of the colon the caecum may perforate

973. **Carcinoma of the lip**
    A   if occurring at the angle of the mouth, tends to be more malignant in behaviour than carcinoma of the upper or lower lip
    B   may be confused with a keratoacanthoma
    C   is curable by surgery
    D   is radioresistant
    E   carries a 40% five-year survival rate if seen in its early stages

974. **A depressed fractured malar bone and zygomatic arch**
    A   may cause diplopia
    B   may cause anaesthesia of the cheek
    C   may cause a palpable notch of the infraorbital margin
    D   is treated conservatively
    E   if compound, is reduced with Walsham's forceps

975. **The overall 5-year and 10-year results of the treatment of carcinoma of the breast are survivals of about**
    A   Stage I 70% cases (5 years)
    B   Stage II 35% cases (5 years)
    C   Stage III 30% cases (5 years)
    D   Stage III 15% cases (10 years)
    E   Stage IV 2% cases (5 years)

976. **Haemorrhage after a child has returned from the theatre for tonsillectomy**
   A is secondary haemorrhage
   B requires that the child should be nursed in the supine position
   C is an indication for an opiate to be given to reduce restlessness
   D requires that grouping and crossmatching of blood should be instituted if simple evacuation of clot and pressure with a swab fails
   E does not mean that a return to the operating theatre may be necessary

977. **In a malignant tumour of the nasopharynx Trotter's triad includes**
   A persistent nasal catarrh
   B epistaxis
   C pain in the side of the head
   D elevation of the homolateral soft palate
   E conductive deafness

978. **The management of a patient with a fractured base of skull includes**
   A propping up the patient to lower pressure and diminish the escape of cerebrospinal fluid
   B incising the suboccipital region if bruising and a boggy swelling in the nape of the neck or below the mastoid process suggests a posterior fossa fracture
   C withholding antibiotics until signs of infection are present
   D finding out if an aerocoele is present
   E early repair of a dural gap

979. **Concerning lung abscess:**
   A The patient may have swallowed a tooth after extraction
   B It is commonly due to aspiration pneumonia
   C The treatment is a combination of chemotherapy and lobectomy
   D It is a cause of cerebral abscess
   E External drainage is never performed today

980. Regarding subarachnoid haemorrhage:
A Prodromal symptoms are common
B There may be comparatively mild headache for a few days before the rupture
C An important premonitory sign is unilateral third nerve palsy presenting as ptosis
D Lumbar puncture must not be done
E A ruptured berry aneurysm requires emergency excision and a Dacron artery replacement under microsurgical control

981. Traumatic intraspinal haemorrhage due to spinal trauma is manifested by
A haematomyelia which is extradural haemorrhage
B haematorrachis which is haemorrhage within the cord
C extradural haemorrhage causing Thorburn's gravitational paraplegia
D immediate paralysis due to haematomyelia
E delayed signs, *e.g.* muscle wasting

982. A carcinoma of the sinus piriformis
A occurs chiefly in women
B causes pain at the onset
C causes pain in the ear
D spreads slowly to involve lymph nodes
E is first treated by excision biopsy

983. Concerning injuries to the eye:
A The pain and photophobia caused by arc welding flash is due to ultraviolet radiation
B Alkali burns are not serious and respond to simple irrigation
C A contusion of the eye may cause a vitreous haemorrhage known as a hyphaema
D Laceration of the eyelids with bleeding coming from beneath the lids suggests the possibility of a perforating eye injury
E An injured eye may have to be enucleated to prevent sympathetic ophthalmia

984. Regarding cleft lip and cleft palate:
A The condition is familial in about 12% of cases
B Clefts on the left greatly outnumber those on the right
C Cleft lip interferes with feeding
D Cleft palate interferes with the patient's ability to learn to speak vowels
E 50% of children with cleft palate have some degree of deafness

985. Regarding laryngeal paralysis:
- A All the muscles of the larynx are innervated by the recurrent laryngeal nerves
- B Routine laryngoscopy of patients reveals that 3–5% have a paresis or paralysis of one vocal cord
- C In 30% of cases no cause can be found
- D Unilateral recurrent nerve paralysis causes a hoarse voice
- E In bilateral recurrent nerve paralysis due to thyroidectomy the cords get sucked together on inspiration and intubation or tracheostomy is essential

986. A patient who is suspected of having an intrabronchial foreign body
- A may have symptoms due to atelectasis
- B may be symptomless
- C may have an x-ray of chest which does not show the foreign body
- D should always be bronchoscoped
- E should wait until inflammation has subsided before removal is attempted

987. In fracture of the os calcis:
- A It is caused by falls from a height
- B The bone is shattered like an eggshell
- C The subtalar joint is spared
- D The heel is everted
- E Anatomical restoration by the use of special compression apparatus gives a good functional result

988. Stricture of the lower end of the oesophagus can be treated by
- A regular dilatation
- B two-thirds polya gastrectomy
- C vagotomy and pyloroplasty
- D Thal's patch
- E Heller's operation

989. The care of a patient immediately after tracheostomy requires
- A the presence of a special nurse
- B that the suction catheters need only to be rinsed and wiped before re-use
- C a trolley beside the bed carrying a fibreoptic E.R.C.P. instrument
- D removal of the tube so the patient is able to sleep
- E that a tracheal dilator is kept beside the patient

990. Ischaemic colitis
- A usually affects the caecum and ascending colon
- B may follow insertion of an aortofemoral prosthesis for an abdominal aneurysm
- C can occur in Buerger's disease (thromboangiitis obliterans)
- D can occur in atherosclerosis
- E should be treated by steroids

991. A localised mass in the right iliac fossa, thought to be due to appendicitis, yet with the patient in a satisfactory condition
- A requires appendicectomy forthwith
- B should be treated conservatively with light diet, analgesics and mild intestinal evacuants
- C should be explored in children
- D should be explored in patients over 65 years
- E is an indication for long term oral antibiotics to be started

992. In the operation of menisectomy
- A the incision is preceded by the application of an Esmarch type of bandage and inflatable tourniquet
- B the incision used for the approach to the medial cartilage is parallel and close to the ligamentum patellae
- C the cartilage is seized and can easily be avulsed
- D a Robert Jones bandage is applied after the incision has been closed and before the tourniquet is released
- E a Robert Jones bandage is an elastic bandage applied just around the knee to cover the patella and the line of the knee joint

993. **Regarding the treatment of carcinoma of the oesophagus:**
    A Gastrostomy is a useful palliative procedure
    B Radiotherapy is most useful in the treatment of squamous cell tumours
    C Growths of the upper third are best treated by surgical extirpation
    D Growths of the lower third are best treated by excision utilising a right thoracic as well as an abdominal approach
    E Columnar-celled tumours are radiosensitive

994. **Regarding operations for hypertrophic pyloric stenosis of infants:**
    A Heller's operation is to be preferred
    B Perforation of the duodenum at operation is fatal
    C Hypothermia is a useful adjunct to the operation
    D In cases complicated by infection of the mouth, operation should take second place to medical treatment
    E Breast fed babies are likely to do better than bottle fed babies because gastroenteritis is a real problem

995. **In fracture of the mandible:**
    A Obtaining correct occlusion is of secondary importance in management
    B An interdental splint can be used
    C Teeth on each side of the fracture should be extracted
    D It is a 'closed' fracture
    E Delayed union is uncommon

996. **A patient with achalasia of the cardia**
    A may present with bronchopneumonia
    B may get a sigmoid oesophagus
    C complains of dysphagia to solids before liquids
    D is unlikely ever to have a carcinoma at the cardia
    E is with advantage operated on through a thoracic approach

997. **To reduce the mechanism of an ankle injury the key is the radiological appearance of the fibular fracture:**
    A Low transverse = inversion injury usually
    B High in the shaft = eversion injury
    C Spiral at the level of the inferior tibiofibular joint = internal rotation injury
    D High transverse = external rotation injury
    E Low transverse = transverse shear

998. Avulsion of the first dorsal nerve root
- A occurs in the case of a falling person clutching at an object and hyperabducting the arm
- B causes paralysis of the intrinsic muscles of the hand
- C causes anaesthesia of all the fingers but not the thumb
- D is likely to cause a Horner's syndrome
- E may be the cause of some spasticity of the leg on the same side

999. The membrana reuniens
- A is the frenum of the tongue
- B is synonymous with the ligament of Treitz
- C is a congenital membrane of the hymen
- D is a fibrous band connecting the skin to the spinal theca
- E may be associated with the appearance of enuresis

1000. When faecal impaction occurs it
- A causes absolute constipation
- B is manifest by the passage of flatus but not faeces
- C is suspected when it is reported that an elderly patient has faecal incontinence or diarrhoea
- D causes abdominal pain and faeces may be palpable through the abdominal wall
- E usually requires disimpaction with the aid of fingers or a tablespoon

1001. The clinical features of acute appendicitis
- A typically begin with vomiting
- B always include pain and tenderness in the right iliac fossa
- C include a rising pulse rate as the condition progresses
- D include hyperpyrexia
- E include pain on coughing

PART V
HISTORICAL. SINGLE RESPONSE 1 IN 4 IN SERIES

This type of question is not as a rule used in any assessments or examinations in surgery. Here they have been set to provide not only a degree of entertainment but to stimulate the student to take an interest in the history of surgery and those giants of the past on whose shoulders we stand today. It is hoped that these questions will stimulate further reading and revision and generally help to fill out the clinical knowledge of any student.

PART V. HISTORICAL

1. **Which of the following is untrue about Mr. Hamilton Bailey?**
   A His father began as a medical missionary in Turkish Palestine
   B He nearly met the same fate as Nurse Cavell in the 1914-18 war
   C His experience of war surgery began at the time of the Battle of Jutland
   D He lost his right little finger as the result of sepsis and this facilitated the performance of a certain clinical examination

2. **Which of the following is untrue about Mr. McNeill Love?**
   A He believed in 'doing today's work today'
   B As a junior hospital doctor he bought a plot of land with his savings so that youth clubs in the east end of London might have a place for recreation
   C He served in Mesopotamia (now Iraq) during the 1914-1918 war
   D He was a Scotsman

3. **In which of the four hospitals that Joseph Lister worked was he not a Professor of Surgery?**
   A University College Hospital, London
   B King's College Hospital, London
   C The Royal Infirmary, Glasgow
   D The Royal Infirmary, Edinburgh

4. **Lord Lister was born in**
   A Edinburgh, Scotland
   B Glasgow, Scotland
   C London, England
   D Peking, China

5. **Lord Lister's first publication on the success of his new treatment of compound fractures and abscesses appeared in**
   A 1865
   B 1867
   C 1870
   D 1874

6. **Which of the following is incorrect about Louis Pasteur in Paris?**
   A He was Professor of Medicine
   B He was a chemist
   C He worked on the isomerism of tartaric acid
   D A shepherd boy was the subject of one of his great experiments

7. **Dominique Larrey was the famous surgeon in Napoleon's army who introduced**
   A internal fixation of fractures
   B debridement
   C delayed primary suture
   D split skin grafting

8. **Which of the following is incorrect about Alexander Fleming (1881-1955)?**
   A He passed the F.R.C.S. examination
   B He worked at St. Mary's Hospital Medical School, London
   C He discovered the penicillium fungus
   D He was a Scotsman

9. **He described the classical clinical features of inflammation**
   A Hippocrates
   B Celsus
   C Menelaus
   G Galen

10. **Oliver Cromwell, Lord Protector of England from 1653-1658, used to insist that his portraits should show him**
    A only in profile
    B head only
    C always wearing a hat
    D wart and all

11. **Which of the following is incorrect about syphilis?**
    A It was brought back by Sir Francis Drake from South America
    B It features in a poem by Girolamo Fracastoro
    C It is called after a shepherd boy named Syphilus
    D It was brought back from Haiti by Christopher Columbus

12. **With one exception Sir William Leishman is associated with**
    A   Delhi boil
    B   the Royal Army Medical Corps
    C   the stain used in haematology
    D   a bacterium named after him

13. **Johann von Esmarch is remembered for the development of**
    A   'flying ambulances' in the battle of Waterloo
    B   the Red Cross
    C   a rubber bandage to act as a tourniquet during the Franco-Prussian war
    D   a blood transfusion apparatus during the 1914–1918 war

14. **He was a physician for a time in Aleppo, Syria, and later became naturalist to the East India Company. He produced a memoir on poisonous snakes in 1787. He was**
    A   Percivall Pott
    B   Patrick Russell
    C   John Abernethy
    D   Joseph Banks

15. **A pioneer neurosurgeon who invented a mixture of beeswax and almond oil to staunch bleeding from the diploe died during the 1914–1918 war in Mesopotamia (Iraq). He was**
    A   Sir Rickman Godlee
    B   Harvey Cushing
    C   Sir William Thorburn
    D   Sir Victor Horsley

16. **Christmas disease (haemophilia B) is so called because**
    A   it was discovered at Christmas time in 1931
    B   it was the name of the patient in whom the disease was discovered
    C   it was the surname of the haematologist who described it
    D   it was first reported from Bethlehem

17. Broadly speaking he spans the period between the death of John Hunter and Lord Lister's discovery of the antiseptic principle. He introduced the words 'electrolyte' and 'anion' and 'cation'
   A Andre Ampère
   B Michael Faraday
   C Allesandro Volta
   D George Ohm

18. Which statement is incorrect concerning Professor J. B. Murphy?
   A He was Professor of Surgery at Jervis Street Hospital, Dublin
   B A biography about him is entitled 'Surgeon Extraordinary'
   C He introduced continuous rectal infusion
   D He invented metal buttons which were used for intestinal anastomosis

19. Why are the words anthrax and carbuncle related?
   A They are conditions which are both caused by the anthrax bacillus
   B Because the common underlying factor is diabetes
   C because they are conditions which only occur on the back of the neck
   D because the ancients likened the conditions to flowing charcoal – carbunculus in Latin; anthrax in Greek

20. William Cobbett called London 'the great wen', but who was the royal personage of that time who had a great wen removed by Sir Astley Cooper in 1821?
   A Queen Anne
   B King George III
   C King George IV
   D Queen Charlotte

21. John Wolfe described full thickness skin graft in 1885. He was
   A a plastic surgeon in Vienna
   B an orthopaedic surgeon in Basle
   C a paediatric surgeon in Quebec
   D an ophthalmic surgeon in Glasgow

22. **Which statement is incorrect about John Hunter (1728–1793), surgeon to St. George's Hospital, London?**
    A He made the voyage to Australia with Captain Cook in order to collect natural history specimens
    B His wife, Anne, wrote an original English libretto for Haydn's 'Creation'
    C He demonstrated the development of collateral circulation
    D He was a pioneer in the teaching of what are now called the basic medical sciences and the setting up of medical schools

23. **Which condition is Jean Charcot of Paris not associated with?**
    A hereditary ataxia
    B peroneal muscular atrophy
    C jaundice
    D tabetic arthropathy

24. **The tendo Achilles is named after Achilles because**
    A he suffered from talipes and had the first ever tendon lengthening operation performed on him
    B he ruptured the tendon in the Olympic games
    C he was bitten there by a snake and died
    D it was the only place in the body where he could be fatally wounded

25. **Only one of the following Professors of Surgery was not a Dublin surgeon and whose name is not connected with fractures about the wrist**
    A Robert Smith
    B Edward Bennett
    C Abraham Colles
    D James Syme

26. **Percival Pott, who described a type of external rotation fracture of the ankle, broke his own leg on the south bank of the Thames. He**
    A was carried between two horses to St. Thomas's Hospital
    B was put in a carriage and taken across London Bridge to St. Bartholomew's Hospital
    C bought a door and had himself carried on this to St. Bartholomew's Hospital
    D hired a passing hearse to take him to Guy's Hospital

195

27. He never held a hospital appointment but is regarded as the founder of orthopaedic surgery
   A Nikolai Pirogoff
   B Sir Robert Jones
   C Hugh Owen Thomas
   D John Howship

28. Marius Smith-Petersen, who introduced the triflanged nail in 1931, was Professor of Orthopaedic Surgery in
   A Stockholm
   B Oslo
   C Toronto
   D Boston

29. With Lord Moynihan, this professor founded the British Journal of Surgery
   A Charles Pannet of St. Mary's Hospital
   B Charles Gask of St. Bartholomew's Hospital
   C William Choyce of University College Hospital
   D Ernest Hey Groves of Bristol Royal Infirmary

30. He introduced cerebral arteriography in 1927 and leucotomy in 1936
   A Antonio Moniz of Lisbon
   B Mirizzi of Buenos Aires
   C Harvey Cushing of Baltimore and Boston
   D Claude Coleman of Richmond, Virginia

31. The man who made the drawings of the circle of arteries at the base of the brain was
   A Thomas Willis, physician
   B John Hunter, surgeon
   C Sir Christopher Wren, architect
   D Leonardo da Vinci, artist, inventor

32. He published 'An Essay on the Shaking Palsy' being
   A a physician in Edinburgh
   B a surgeon in Dublin
   C a neurologist in Boston
   D a general practitioner in London

33. He discovered pepsin and was the first to recognise the cell as the unit of living tissue. Much of his original work was done before the age of 27
   A   Theodore Schwann (Louvain and Liège)
   B   Wilhelm Erb (Heidelberg)
   C   Johann Lieberkühn (Berlin)
   D   Johann Brunner (Basle)

34. He described a position for pelvic operations in 1890
   A   Charles Denonvilliers
   B   James Douglas
   C   Friedrich Trendelenburg
   D   Johann Pfannenstiel

35. To get rid of a foreign body in the ear he recommended tying the patient on to a wooden plank with the ear downwards and hitting the plank with a hammer
   A   Prosper Menière of Paris
   B   Aulus Celsus of Rome 25 B.C.–50 A.D.
   C   Nathaniel Highmore of Sherborne, Dorset
   D   Bartolomeo Eustachi of San Severino, Italy

36. Leonardo Gigli of Florence, Italy, invented his wire saw in 1894 particularly for
   A   craniotomy
   B   mandibulectomy
   C   intertrochanteric osteotomy
   D   pubiotomy

37. He abandoned medicine (after, it is said, failing to get a particular anatomy post), became a bishop and is regarded as the father of geology
   A   John Hunter of London
   B   Thomas Wharton of London
   C   Philipp Passavant of Frankfurt
   D   Niels Stensen of Copenhagen

38. Which of the following is not associated with the foundation of a clinic in the U.S.A.?
   A   George Crile
   B   Frank Lahey
   C   William Mayo
   D   Caleb Parry

39. Where did Pythia the snake woman oracle sit on her tripod clutching the monolithic 'omphalos' of the world?
    A   Athens
    B   Epidaurus
    C   Delphi
    D   Mycenae

40. Which is the odd man out?
    A   Carl von Basedow of Merseberg, Germany
    B   Caleb Hillier Parry of Bath, England
    C   Sir William Gull of London
    D   Robert Graves of Dublin

41. He was the first to use iodine for preparing thyrotoxic patients for operation
    A   Jean Lugol of Paris
    B   Henry Plummer of Rochester, Minn., U.S.A.
    C   Sir Thomas Dunhill of London
    D   William Halsted of Baltimore

42. The concept of Hashimoto's disease as an auto-immune thyroiditis was defined in 1956 by
    A   Fritz de Quervain of Berne
    B   Bernhard Riedet and colleagues of Jeva
    C   Charles Huggins and colleagues of Chicago
    D   Ivan Roitt and colleagues of London

43. Rupert Waterhouse of Bath, England, and Carl Friderichson of Copenhagen described the now eponymous syndrome respectively in
    A   1911 and 1918
    B   1931 and 1938
    C   1951 and 1958
    D   1961 and 1968

44. What did Sir Astley Cooper of Guy's Hospital, London, describe in 1829?
    A   Chimney sweeps' cancer
    B   the ligament on the brim of the pelvis
    C   scrofulous swellings in the bosoms of young women
    D   how he removed the sebaceous cyst from the head of King George IV

45. Oophorectomy for breast cancer was described in 1896 by George Beatson. He worked in
    A Glasgow
    B London
    C Montreal
    D New York

46. Which of the following innovations was William Halsted of Baltimore not associated with?
    A Radical mastectomy
    B Rubber operating gloves
    C Local anaesthetics
    D Cholecystostomy

47. The first to carry out adrenalectomy successfully (and a Nobel Prize Winner) was
    A Charles Huggins of Chicago
    B Carl Semb of Oslo
    C Clarence Crafoord of Stockholm
    D Rudolph Matas of New Orleans

48. Dr. Davis of Boston invented it and Dr. Boyle of London (St. Bartholomew's Hospital) improved it. It is
    A an endotracheal tube
    B an adenoid curette
    C a type of post-nasal pack
    D a mouth gag used for tonsillectomy

49. Professor Chevalier Jackson was
    A a pioneer in broncho-oesophagoscopy from Philadelphia
    B one of the founders of anaesthetics from Boston
    C a mediastinoscopist from Paris
    D the first British surgeon to perform a thoracoplasty

50. What did Professor Joe Meigs of Boston, U.S.A., describe?
    A a method of laparoscopy
    B rib resection for empyaema
    C a syndrome to do with ovarian fibroma
    D a test for diabetes mellitis

51. He described an operation in 1908 which was first performed successfully in 1942 by Kirschner
   A James Roberts and mitral valvotomy
   B Friedrich Trendelenburg and pulmonary embolectomy
   C Arthur Hassall and thymectomy
   D Ernst Sauerbruch and lobectomy

52. What was the first successful operation that Alfred Blalock of John Hopkins University performed in 1939
   A for Fallots tetralogy
   B Thymectomy for myaesthenia gravis
   C Porta-caval anastomosis
   D Mitral valvotomy

53. Sir Dominic Corrigan, who described the water hammer pulse in 1832 was
   A a surgeon in Gibraltar
   B a physician in Malta
   C a physician in Dublin
   D a surgeon in Quebec

54. Rudolph Nissen of the Nissen fundoplication operation for hiatus hernia held two chairs of surgery in succession. They were in
   A Leipzig and Vienna
   B Vienna and Innsbruck
   C Trieste and Strasbourg
   D Istanbul and Basle

55. Paterson and Kelly described in 1919 the syndrome also described by Plummer and Vinson in 1921. Paterson and Kelly were British
   A general surgeons
   B physicians
   C otorhinolaryngologists
   D radiologists

56. Noteworthy in the history and practice of gastric surgery he altered the spelling of his name when he discovered his grandfather had mis-spelt it
   A Christian Billroth
   B Berkeley Moynihan
   C William Mayo
   D Wilhelm Ramstedt

57. **Thomas Blizard Curling of The London Hospital described in 1842**
    A a game to be played on the ice
    B a stress ulcer of the duodenum after burns
    C frostbite syndrome
    D a contracture of the hand following a scald

58. **Eugen Polya of gastrectomy fame was a surgeon in**
    A Belgrade
    B Budapest
    C Vienna
    D Trieste

59. **Einar Meulengracht who introduced in 1934 early liberal puree feeding of a bleeding peptic ulcer was**
    A Dutch
    B Danish
    C Belgian
    D German

60. **He diagnosed his own gastric cancer by his own sign**
    A Armand Trousseau
    B Charles Troisier
    C Bernard Naunyn
    D Thomas Cullen

61. **Galen was personal physician to the Roman Emperor**
    A Hadrian
    B Commodus
    C Antoninus (Caracalla)
    D Severus Alexander

62. **Gregor Mendel whose work on inheritance in 1866 passed almost unnoticed during his life time was**
    A a naturalist of Uppsala, Sweden
    B the father of the German composer
    C a Russian chemist
    D an Augustinian monk

63. **He practised in Formosa and Hong Kong and is regarded as the 'Father of Tropical Medicine'**
    A William Leishman
    B Ronald Ross
    C Patrick Manson
    D Theodor Bilharz

64. **George Budd who was probably the first to describe the Budd-Chiari syndrome**
    A was a surgeon to the Royal Navy
    B was the subject of a story by Herman Melville
    C became Governor-General of Canada
    D was Professor of Medicine at King's College Hospital, London

65. **He described a type of cirrhosis and he invented the stethoscope in 1819**
    A Francis Glisson
    B Victor Hanot
    C Tommaso Casoni
    D Rene Laennec

66. **Francis Glisson who described the capsule of the liver was**
    A Professor of Surgery in Paris
    B Regius Professor of Physic in Cambridge
    C Professor of Anatomy in Padua
    D an anatomist of Basle

67. **He was murdered when entering his house at night**
    A Ruggero Oddi of Perugia
    B Antonio Scarpa of Pavia
    C Johann Wirsung of Padua
    D Abraham Vater of Wittenberg

68. **Cholecystography was discovered incidentally by Graham and Cole when they were young as**
    A radiologists
    B a physician and a radiologist
    C a surgeon and a physician
    D surgeons

69. **He said that a gallstone is a tombstone erected to the memory of the organism within it**
    A Eugene du Bois
    B Mecker von Hemsbach
    C Harvey Cushing
    D Berkeley Moynihan

70. **The Phrygian cap**
    A was worn exclusively by virgins in the French Revolution
    B refers to hats worn by a people in Asia Minor
    C was worn by pirates
    D is the curved end of a cystoscope

71. He used to teach about but did not himself publish the triad of gallstones, diverticulosis and hiatus hernia
    A   Jean Charcot of Paris
    B   Jonathan Hutchinson of London
    C   Ludwig Courvoisier of Basle
    D   Charles Saint of Cape Town

72. In an attack of biliary colic 'he called his family and, bidding them farewell, turned his face to the wall to await death. Nevertheless, next morning he was up betimes and in fair spirits'. He was
    A   Lord Moynihan
    B   Robert Browning
    C   Sir Walter Scott
    D   John Hunter

73. Murphy's sign is also known as
    A   Moynihan's test
    B   Naunyn's sign
    C   Courvoisier's law
    D   Petit's triad

74. Typhoid Mary was
    A   an Australian housewife
    B   a Scottish barmaid
    C   a New York cook
    D   a London lavatory attendant

75. A distinguished Professor of Surgery, Basle, Switzerland, made a statement about the probability of a distended gall bladder in jaundiced cases
    A   Fritz de Quervain
    B   Rudolph Nissen
    C   Emil Kocher
    D   Ludwig Courvoisier

76. Allen Oldfather Whipple was a Professor of Surgery in
    A   New York
    B   Toronto
    C   Dublin
    D   Edinburgh

77. **Hippocrates was born**
    A at Epidaurus
    B in Crete
    C in Cos
    D in Delos

78. **He was Major General of the Royal Army Medical Service and described Malta fever in 1887**
    A Sir William Leishman
    B Sir David Bruce
    C Lord Moynihan
    D Philip Mitchiner

79. **He was the first to perform deliberate appendicectomy for acute appendicitis in May, 1880. The patient recovered**
    A Charles McBurney of New York
    B David Wilkie of Edinburgh
    C Heber Fitz of Boston
    D Lawson Tait of Birmingham

80. **The first recorded operation for an appendix abscess in 1848 was by**
    A Sir Frederick Treves of The London Hospital
    B Lawson Tait of the Queen's Hospital, Birmingham
    C Robert Liston of University College Hospital, London
    D Henry Hancock of Charing Cross Hospital, London

81. **Of ischiorectal renown he was dismissed from his post for a breach of the Anatomy Act and disappeared in America. (Might his spirit have returned by air?)**
    A Benjamin Alcock of Cork
    B James Douglas of London
    C Charles Bent Ball of Dublin
    D John Houston of Dublin

82. **Known as the 'first English surgeon' (14th century) he practised in Norwich**
    A Sir Thomas Browne
    B John of Arderne
    C Richard Wiseman
    D John of Gaddesden

83. **For successfully treating Louis XIV's fistula-in-ano he received 300,000 livres**
    A   John of Arderne
    B   Frère Jacques
    C   Charles Félix
    D   Charles Roux

84. **This hospital in London was founded in 1835 for the treatment of anal fistula**
    A   St. Mary's
    B   St. Mark's
    C   St. John's
    D   St. Luke's

85. **He was a comparative anatomist and conservator of the Hunterian Museum of the Royal College of Surgeons of England**
    A   George Ellis
    B   John of Arderne
    C   Cuthbert Dukes
    D   Arthur Keith

86. **Coudé in urology refers to**
    A   a French surgeon, François Coudé who invented a catheter
    B   a French rubber technician who made Jaques' catheter
    C   a catheter with an angled bend near the tip
    D   a bougie with an angled bend near the tip

87. **He and Benechey, an optician in Vienna, produced the first cystoscope in 1877**
    A   Frère Jacques
    B   Achille Malecot
    C   Theodor Bilharz
    D   Max Nitze

88. **The lithotomy position is so called because**
    A   it means, literally, to lie on the back with the legs apart and knees bent
    B   it is the position used by athletes when resting after a race
    C   it means literally 'opening between the buttocks'
    D   it was the position used for removal of stones from the bladder

89. Frère Jacques was
   A   a French surgeon
   B   a French physician
   C   an Italian serving in the French army
   D   an Italian priest but also a surgeon

90. He was a director of the first school of art as applied to medicine
   A   Max Brödel
   B   Theodor Klebs
   C   Max Wilms
   D   Alexander Borodin

91. Frère Jacques performed lithotomy with
   A   an amputation knife
   B   a Gigli saw
   C   a bread knife
   D   a pruning knife

92. He was the first to succeed in closing a vesico-vaginal fistula
   A   Lawson Tait, surgeon of Birmingham, United Kingdom
   B   Guy Hunner, gynaecologist of Baltimore
   C   Johann Diffenbach, surgeon of Berlin
   D   James Marion Sims, while a country practitioner of Alabama

93. The association between bladder tumours and anilene dyes was first suspected by
   A   Francis Kidd of London in 1924
   B   Ludwig Rehn of Germany in 1894
   C   Theodor Bilharz of Cairo in 1861
   D   Guy Hunner of Baltimore in 1930

94. He 'discovered' prostatectomy while in the Indian Medical Service
   A   Harry Harris of Sydney
   B   Hugh Young of Baltimore
   C   Henry Bigelow of Boston
   D   Peter Freyer of London

95. Hans Reiter described Reiter's disease in 1916. He was President of the Health Service in
    A South West Africa
    B Berlin
    C Vienna
    D Singapore

96. He bequeathed 13682 museum specimens prepared and mounted by his own hands
    A Percivall Pott of London
    B Giovanni Morgani of Padua
    C John Hunter of London
    D François de la Peyronie of Paris

97. This historian died because his hernia as well as his hydrocoele was punctured by a trochar and cannula
    A Anton Nuck of Leiden
    B Joachim Giraldes of Paris
    C Enrico Sertoli of Milan
    D Edward Gibbon of London

98. Chimney sweeps' cancer was first described in 1775 by
    A John Abernethy, St. Bartholomew's Hospital
    B John Hunter, St. George's Hospital
    C Edward Cock, Guy's Hospital
    D Percivall Pott, St. Bartholomew's Hospital

99. Alexis Carrell who pioneered transplantation worked in
    A Cairo
    B Kuala Lumpur
    C New York
    D Moscow

100. The first human heart transplant in the world was performed in
    A Budapest, 1966
    B Bombay, 1969
    C San Francisco, 1970
    D Cape Town, 1967

101. The Brompton mixture emanates from the Brompton Hospital, London, which is
 A   a district general hospital
 B   a chest hospital
 C   an orthopaedic hospital
 D   a children's hospital

ANSWERS

PART I

1. A	40. B	79. D
2. B	41. D	80. C
3. C	42. D	81. A
4. D	43. C	82. C
5. B	44. C	83. D
6. B	45. C	84. D
7. D	46. D	85. D
8. C	47. D	86. C
9. B	48. B	87. D
10. D	49. C	88. C
11. A	50. A	89. C
12. B	51. D	90. B
13. C	52. C	91. A
14. D	53. C	92. C
15. B	54. C	93. D
16. B	55. B	94. C
17. B	56. C	95. C
18. C	57. C	96. B
19. A	58. C	97. B
20. A	59. D	98. B
21. A	60. C	99. B
22. B	61. C	100. C
23. C	62. D	101. D
24. B	63. C	102. D
25. B	64. D	103. B
26. B	65. C	104. A
27. A	66. B	105. B
28. A	67. C	106. A
29. C	68. B	107. A
30. B	69. C	108. B
31. A	70. D	109. A
32. D	71. A	110. C
33. A	72. D	111. B
34. C	73. B	112. D
35. D	74. D	113. C
36. C	75. B	114. D
37. C	76. A	115. C
38. C	77. C	116. D
39. C	78. C	117. C

118. C	162. C	206. D
119. A	163. C	207. A
120. C	164. B	208. D
121. C	165. D	209. C
122. D	166. B	210. D
123. C	167. A	211. B
124. D	168. D	212. A
125. B	169. A	213. C
126. C	170. B	214. A
127. D	171. A	215. C
128. B	172. B	216. A
129. D	173. A	217. A
130. A	174. A	218. D
131. B	175. B	219. C
132. B	176. B	220. B
133. D	177. D	221. D
134. C	178. D	222. A
135. A	179. A	223. A
136. C	180. B	224. D
137. B	181. D	225. D
138. B	182. B	226. A
139. C	183. D	227. C
140. D	184. C	228. D
141. B	185. D	229. D
142. D	186. C	230. B
143. A	187. A	231. D
144. D	188. B	232. A
145. C	189. A	233. D
146. C	190. A	234. D
147. D	191. A	235. A
148. C	192. D	236. C
149. D	193. A	237. B
150. B	194. B	238. C
151. A	195. D	239. D
152. D	196. D	240. D
153. A	197. C	241. A
154. A	198. C	242. D
155. D	199. B	243. A
156. D	200. A	244. A
157. D	201. D	245. A
158. A	202. D	246. D
159. D	203. D	247. C
160. B	204. B	248. C
161. B	205. D	249. D

250. D	267. D	284. C
251. B	268. A	285. A
252. C	269. B	286. C
253. D	270. A	287. D
254. D	271. D	288. D
255. A	272. D	289. D
256. B	273. C	290. D
257. A	274. A	291. A
258. C	275. D	292. B
259. A	276. B	293. A
260. D	277. D	294. D
261. A	278. C	295. C
262. C	279. D	296. D
263. B	280. A	297. D
264. A	281. C	298. B
265. A	282. C	299. C
266. B	283. A	300. C

PART II

301. A C E
302. A B D
303. A D
304. D E
305. B
306. C D
307. A D E
308. B C
309. A C D
310. A B E
311. C E
312. B C D E
313. A B
314. A C D
315. B D E
316. E
317. A C D E
318. None
319. A B C
320. A B C D E
321. C D E
322. C D E
323. A B C
324. B C E
325. A D E
326. B D E
327. A C D
328. D E
329. B
330. A B C
331. B D
332. C D
333. A B C D E
334. A B C D E
335. A B C
336. D E
337. E
338. D
339. None

340. D E
341. C E
342. A E
343. E
344. B C D
345. B C E
346. A C D
347. D E
348. A B
349. B C E
350. A B C
351. A B E
352. A B C
353. B C
354. A B C D
355. B C
356. C D E
357. C
358. C E
359. A B D
360. B E
361. B C
362. A B C
363. A B C
364. A B C D
365. A B C D
366. A B
367. A C D
368. A E
369. A B C D E
370. A B C
371. B
372. C D
373. A E
374. A D E
375. A C E
376. A B E
377. A D E
378. B C D

379. None
380. A B E
381. A B C D
382. B D E
383. C D E
384. B D
385. B D E
386. A C E
387. B C D E
388. A
389. C D E
390. None
391. A B C
392. A C E
393. A D E
394. A
395. A B E
396. C D
397. C E
398. A B C
399. A B C D E
400. A C D E
401. B E
402. E
403. A B C
404. A B C D E
405. A B C
406. B D
407. B C
408. A B
409. C D
410. A D
411. A C D E
412. A B C D
413. A B
414. B D
415. B C D
416. A C D
417. A D E

418. B E	462. D	506. B E
419. C E	463. B D E	507. A B D
420. D	464. B C D	508. A B C
421. A	465. None	509. A B E
422. C D	466. A B C	510. A D
423. C	467. A D	511. A C D
424. A D	468. B D	512. D E
425. B C D E	469. A C E	513. C D
426. A B C	470. C D	514. D E
427. A C E	471. A C D E	515. A B D
428. A B C D	472. C D E	516. B
429. B D E	473. D E	517. A B
430. A B C D	474. C D	518. A B C D
431. A B E	475. D E	519. B C
432. A D E	476. A C	520. B C D
433. B D	477. A B C D	521. A
434. C D	478. D E	522. B C D
435. A B D	479. A D	523. A E
436. A B C D E	480. A C D	524. B D E
437. B E	481. D E	525. C E
438. A E	482. A B D	526. B C D
439. C E	483. D E	527. A C D E
440. A B E	484. A B C D	528. B
441. C	485. C	529. B D E
442. A C D E	486. A C D	530. B C E
443. D E	487. A D E	531. C E
444. D E	488. C D E	532. None
445. A B C	489. C E	533. B C D
446. A B C D E	490. B C	534. A E
447. B C E	491. A B C	535. D
448. A B E	492. A B E	536. B C D E
449. B C D	493. A E	537. B C E
450. B C E	494. A E	538. C D E
451. D	495. None	539. B C D E
452. A C D	496. C D	540. A B C
453. A B C D E	497. A B C D E	541. D E
454. A C D	498. A B C	542. B D
455. A B C E	499. A	543. A B C
456. A B C E	500. B C D	544. A C D E
457. A C E	501. A B C	545. A B C D E
458. E	502. A C D	546. A
459. B C E	503. B D	547. B C E
460. A C E	504. A B C E	548. B C D
461. A B C	505. A B	549. A B C D E

550. A C	567. A B C D E	584. A D E
551. C E	568. A B C	585. A E
552. D	569. D E	586. B C
553. B E	570. A B C D	587. A B C
554. A B	571. A B	588. A D E
555. A D	572. A B C	589. D E
556. D	573. A C D E	590. B C
557. A B C	574. B C E	591. B D E
558. B C D	575. None	592. C E
559. C D	576. C D	593. B C E
560. A C	577. A B E	594. D E
561. A B C D	578. C D E	595. A B E
562. A	579. C D E	596. D E
563. A B C D E	580. C E	597. A C E
564. B C D	581. A C	598. A B D E
565. A B E	582. E	599. None
566. A B C D E	583. A B C D	600. A E

PART III

601. D	640. C	679. A
602. D	641. D	680. D
603. C	642. A	681. A
604. B	643. C	682. C
605. C	644. A	683. D
606. C	645. C	684. D
607. A	646. B	685. C
608. C	647. C	686. D
609. C	648. A	687. C
610. A	649. C	688. D
611. D	650. A	689. C
612. A	651. D	690. D
613. C	652. A	691. D
614. B	653. C	692. D
615. B	654. D	693. B
616. A	655. D	694. D
617. C	656. A	695. D
618. C	657. D	696. A
619. C	658. C	697. A
620. D	659. A	698. D
621. C	660. A	699. D
622. C	661. C	700. C
623. B	662. C	701. C
624. A	663. C	702. B
625. D	664. D	703. C
626. B	665. B	704. C
627. A	666. B	705. A
628. A	667. C	706. C
629. A	668. C	707. D
630. D	669. B	708. C
631. A	670. C	709. A
632. B	671. C	710. C
633. C	672. D	711. A
634. A	673. B	712. C
635. D	674. D	713. A
636. A	675. C	714. C
637. D	676. B	715. D
638. C	677. D	716. C
639. D	678. D	717. C

718. B	746. B	774. A
719. D	747. D	775. A
720. D	748. B	776. B
721. C	749. D	777. B
722. B	750. D	778. C
723. C	751. C	779. C
724. B	752. B	780. C
725. C	753. D	781. C
726. D	754. D	782. C
727. D	755. C	783. B
728. C	756. A	784. D
729. B	757. A	785. A
730. D	758. C	786. B
731. B	759. C	787. C
732. D	760. C	788. B
733. A	761. B	789. C
734. A	762. D	790. D
735. D	763. D	791. C
736. D	764. D	792. C
737. C	765. A	793. A
738. A	766. B	794. C
739. A	767. D	795. C
740. B	768. C	796. A
741. C	769. D	797. A
742. C	770. B	798. D
743. B	771. C	799. C
744. C	772. A	800. D
745. B	773. A	

PART IV

801. A B D
802. C E
803. A B C
804. A C E
805. A C D
806. C D
807. A B
808. None
809. C D E
810. B C D
811. D E
812. C D E
813. B C
814. C D
815. A B E
816. B C E
817. A B D
818. A B D
819. A C D
820. A B C E
821. C D E
822. A B
823. C D
824. A B C
825. B C E
826. B D
827. A C D E
828. A B D
829. A B D
830. A C E
831. B C
832. A C
833. C D
834. A B E
835. C D E
836. B D
837. B C
838. A E
839. A B C E
840. B D
841. A E
842. A B C D E
843. B D E
844. C D
845. A B E
846. A C E
847. C D
848. B C E
849. A D E
850. A C
851. A D E
852. A C D
853. C E
854. A D
855. A B
856. C D E
857. B E
858. A B D
859. B C E
860. B C
861. A B E
862. C D E
863. A B C
864. B D E
865. D E
866. B D E
867. A C D
868. A B
869. B D
870. B C
871. B D E
872. A B C D E
873. A E
874. B C D
875. C E
876. A B E
877. A D
878. A B E
879. A C E
880. A B D E
881. A B C D E
882. A C D E
883. A C D
884. C D E
885. A B C
886. A D
887. A B C D E
888. C D E
889. A D E
890. A B C
891. C E
892. B C D
893. A C E
894. A C
895. B C E
896. C
897. C D
898. A B D
899. A E
900. B E
901. A C
902. A
903. A B C
904. A B C
905. A B C D E
906. A B C D
907. B C
908. A B
909. D
910. C D E
911. A B D
912. A D E
913. A D
914. A B C D E
915. B D
916. B C D
917. A B E

918. A C D
919. C E
920. C D
921. A B D
922. A B E
923. A C E
924. B C E
925. B C E
926. A B D
927. C D E
928. B C
929. A B
930. A B E
931. A D
932. A E
933. A B E
934. A B E
935. B C
936. A D E
937. C D
938. A E
939. B E
940. B C E
941. B D
942. B C E
943. A B D
944. B D E
945. E

946. B D E
947. B E
948. C D
949. A B E
950. A B D E
951. B C D
952. A C
953. A B C
954. A B C E
955. A B C D
956. A B C
957. A C
958. B D
959. B C
960. A D
961. B C D
962. B
963. A B C D
964. A B C E
965. B C D
966. A B D
967. A C D
968. A D E
969. A B
970. B C E
971. A C E
972. A B E
973. A B C

974. A B C
975. A B E
976. D
977. C D E
978. A D E
979. B D
980. B C
981. C D E
982. C
983. A D E
984. A B E
985. B C E
986. A B C D
987. A B D
988. A B C D
989. A E
990. B C D
991. C D
992. A D
993. B D
994. D E
995. B
996. A B E
997. A B
998. A B D E
999. D E
1000. C D E
1001. C E

PART V – HISTORICAL

1. D	35. B	69. D
2. D	36. D	70. B
3. A	37. D	71. D
4. C	38. D	72. C
5. B	39. C	73. B
6. A	40. C	74. C
7. B	41. B	75. D
8. C	42. D	76. A
9. B	43. A	77. C
10. D	44. C	78. B
11. A	45. A	79. D
12. D	46. D	80. D
13. C	47. A	81. A
14. B	48. D	82. B
15. D	49. A	83. C
16. B	50. C	84. B
17. B	51. B	85. D
18. A	52. B	86. C
19. D	53. C	87. D
20. C	54. D	88. D
21. D	55. C	89. C
22. A	56. D	90. A
23. A	57. B	91. C
24. D	58. B	92. D
25. D	59. B	93. B
26. C	60. A	94. D
27. C	61. B	95. B
28. D	62. D	96. C
29. D	63. C	97. D
30. A	64. D	98. D
31. C	65. D	99. C
32. D	66. B	100. D
33. A	67. C	101. B
34. C	68. D	